THE ENERGETICS OF HEALTH

Commissioning Editor: Claire Wilson
Development Editor: Veronika Watkins
Project Manager: Anne Dickie and Jagannathan Varadarajan
Designer: Erik Bigland
Illustrators: David Banks (Cover image) and Marion Tasker
Illustration Manager: Kirsteen Wright

THE ENERGETICS OF HEALTH: A NATUROPATHIC ASSESSMENT

Iva Lloyd BScH RPP ND
Chair of CAND, Naturopathic Foundations Health Clinic
Markham, Ontario
Canada

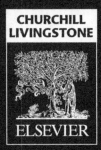

CHURCHILL
LIVINGSTONE

ELSEVIER

EDINBURGH LONDON NEW YORK OXFORD PHILADELPHIA ST LOUIS SYDNEY
TORONTO 2009

CHURCHILL
LIVINGSTONE
ELSEVIER

ISBN: 978-0-443-06955-0

British Library Cataloguing in Publication Data
A catalogue record for this book is available from the British Library

Library of Congress Cataloging in Publication Data
A catalog record for this book is available from the Library of Congress

Notice
Knowledge and best practice in this field are constantly changing. As new research and experience broaden our knowledge, changes in practice, treatment and drug therapy may become necessary or appropriate. Readers are advised to check the most current information provided (i) on procedures featured or (ii) by the manufacturer of each product to be administered, to verify the recommended dose or formula, the method and duration of administration, and contraindications. It is the responsibility of the practitioner, relying on their own experience and knowledge of the patient, to make diagnoses, to determine dosages and the best treatment for each individual patient, and to take all appropriate safety precautions. To the fullest extent of the law, neither the Publisher nor the Editors assumes any liability for any injury and/or damage to persons or property arising out of or related to any use of the material contained in this book.

The Publisher

CONTENTS

SECTION III NATUROPATHIC ASSESSMENT

SECTION IV TREATMENT STRATEGIES

PREFACE

The foundation of this book was created over a 10-year span during which time I taught a course to polarity therapy practitioners on how to conduct an assessment based on energetic principles. The principles used were based on Ayurvedic and Chinese medicine. During that period I was also studying and practicing as a naturopathic doctor. Polarity therapy provided an energetic perspective; naturopathic medicine provided the education and the principles and philosophy that brought it all together.

Human beings have always marveled at the intrinsic and mysterious ability of the body to grow, regenerate and heal. The search for the factors that prevent and cause disease has been the basis of medicine since the beginning of time. Every medical system has its own language and framework for understanding the mysteries of the human body, and these frameworks change and develop over time.

Traditional medical systems were based on observing the interaction of people with their environment and they approach health and disease based on holistic and vitalistic concepts. In contrast, the conventional medical system is based on a dualistic view of the body and mind and a mechanistic approach to studying its inner functions. The naturopathic medical system developed partly out of frustration with the shortcomings of the conventional medical system and it embraces many of the concepts of traditional medical systems, such as a belief in a more vitalistic and holistic approach to health. The founders of naturopathic medicine recognized an inherent ability of the body to heal and they believed that 'wrongful living' was a contributing factor to many diseases, especially chronic disease.

Much of the study of the mystery and meaning of life started in the field of philosophy; with observation and curiosity about the interconnectedness of health and disease with a person's lifestyle and environment. Over time research has become more focused on studying the individual parts, separate from the whole. From a conventional perspective, the causes of disease are often viewed as malfunctioning parts of the body separate from the lifestyle or life experiences of the patient. This narrow perspective ignores the interrelationship of different organ systems, let alone the relationship between human beings and their environment. The view of humans as biochemical beings has resulted in a healthcare system that is based on pharmaceutical agents and substances that patients take in order to address symptoms, versus changes that a patient needs to make.

Over time we have seen a shift in the mindset of patients and practitioners as there is growing knowledge about the detrimental effects of environmental toxins, chemicals and pharmaceuticals. There is increased concern about the health of the environment and the effects all of this will have on future generations. People have a greater insight into the ability of the mind to affect health and to contribute to disease; that structural changes in the body can affect internal functioning that all parts of a person are connected.

Our understanding of the nature of human beings is scattered across different disciplines. Each one holds a piece of the puzzle and provides insight into the mystery of life. The discovery of an electrical field of light energy around every tangible and intangible component of life expands the knowledge and understanding for how communication happens within the body, between individuals, and among individuals and their external environment. Systems theory provides a model for exploring human beings as complex, dynamic systems which have the ability to self-organize and self-renew based on information exchanged internally and externally. What is apparent is that to understand the factors that contribute to health and disease there is a need for communication and collaboration between healthcare providers of various medical traditions and professionals from other disciplines.

THE PURPOSE OF THIS BOOK

The purpose of the book is to provide a model for assessing the causal factors of disease using a framework based on naturopathic principles and the qualities and characteristic patterns that emerge. These patterns manifest in language, in the physical body, in symptoms and in diseases. These same qualities and characteristics correspond to food, nature and all aspects of life; they can be understood at any level – cellular to physical, concrete to conceptual, and physical to emotional. It is easier to discern the causal lifestyle and environmental factors when a common framework and language is used throughout the assessment, diagnosis and treatment process.

The model provided is based on naturopathic principles, concepts common to the traditional medical systems of Ayurvedic, Chinese and Unani medicine, and current theories that support the vitalistic and holistic concepts of naturopathic medicine. It brings together pieces from a number of different systems of medicine and although I do not present incontrovertible evidence to prove the correlation, there is considerable evidence to support this model. There is much research and focus on how the body responds when in a disease state; what is often missing is a focus on the factors that caused the disruption to health, and the belief that the body has an innate ability to heal.

Health and disease is a continuum. A patient's state of health at any point in time is dependent and influenced by many factors, including their inherent constitution, their lifestyle and external factors. Health is the harmonious vibration of all aspects of an individual within themselves and with their external environment. On an ongoing basis the body is continuously responding to, adapting to and compensating for internal and external factors. When these factors overwhelm the homeodynamic state of the body, health is disrupted and symptoms manifest in a way that is meaningful and relates back to the causal factors. The body has an innate ability to heal (*vis medicatrix naturae*) and at times symptoms are a reflection of this innate ability. The aim of naturopathic medicine is to identify and address the factors that are obstructing healing. It involves teaching patients how to live a life that is in balance with their constitution; it is about changing the current model from 'What do I take' to 'What do I do.'

When symptoms or diseases manifest, the focus of many medical systems is to assess the impact that the symptoms are having on health. Although naturopathic medicine also does this, the aim of naturopathic medicine is on identifying the causal factors that are preventing the innate healing ability of the body, to provide the body with the building blocks that it needs for health, and to support this healing ability.

This book provides a naturopathic assessment model aimed at correlating the symptom and disease patterns with their causal factors. The term *assessment* is purposely chosen, versus the term diagnosis. Assessment is the process of observing, listening, analyzing and collecting data from a patient; diagnosis is the identification or labeling of the findings from the assessment. In naturopathic medicine the patient's subjective experience of their symptoms and diseases, and the patient's awareness of the timing and nature of the symptoms are an important part of the assessment. The purpose of an assessment is to identify what a patient needs to change or what they need to address. The accuracy of any diagnosis and the success of a treatment plan depend on the thoroughness of the assessment process and the degree to which the causal factors have been identified.

For any health practitioner, the assessment of health and disease includes addressing a growing number of factors, including lifestyle, mental and emotional, external and environmental factors, and medical. The number of variables that affect health is extensive, and irrespective of the treatment strategy all variables that are having a disrupting effect are best identified and addressed.

OUTLINE OF THE BOOK

This book is broken down into three main sections. The first section starts with a brief look at the changing perspectives of health and disease, from the ancient era to the current postmodern era. To understand and appreciate the advances and the challenges of healthcare it is valuable to have an understanding of its evolution. The traditional systems of medicine, such as Ayurvedic, Chinese and Unani medicine, have been around for thousands of years and have contributed greatly to the holistic and vitalistic approaches to life. They view and explain all aspects of life, health and disease based on the qualities and characteristics that they hold. A brief overview of these systems of medicine is provided as an introduction to looking at aspects of life and disease based on their characteristics and qualities. Naturopathic doctors are trained in the biomedical sciences, yet they also recognize the importance of the patient's 'story', the interrelationship of all aspects of an individual, the role of the patient–practitioner interaction, and the importance of lifestyle and environmental factors on health. What sets the naturopathic medical system apart from the conventional healthcare system is its strong belief in the healing power of nature. There is recognition that health and disease are a continuum that is influenced and determined by various factors. The book reviews the principles and philosophies of naturopathic medicine and provides a detailed naturopathic assessment model that is designed to aid practitioners in identifying the causal factors of disease.

The second section of the book provides an overview of the concepts and theories that are used in the assessment model. It explores humans as energetic beings of light, the intangible and tangible nature of cellular communication, and the importance of water and movement to life. It reviews the theories behind human beings as complex systems such as self-organization, self-renewal and self-transcendence. The qualities and characteristics of the patterns of internal and external, excess and deficiency, Yin–Yang and the five elements are explored as a guide for understanding the link between causal factors and symptoms and diseases. Theories for understanding the transformation between health and disease are also provided. Where available, the research to support the principles and concepts behind these theories and patterns is used. For some of the concepts, there is not the research to substantiate or disprove the theories, yet there is a wealth of historic information to provide a framework for these theories.

The third and largest section of the book provides a detailed look at how to apply these theories and concepts throughout the assessment process. There is an emphasis on the therapeutic encounter and the wealth of information that is conveyed through the patient's recall of their subjective experience. The main aspects of the physical assessment (such as tongue and pulse diagnosis, postural assessment, assessment of the face, and the fingers and toes) that most clearly display the energetic patterns are reviewed in detail. Case studies and examples are used to highlight the key concepts and to provide additional insights into how to apply the information in practice.

ACKNOWLEDGMENTS

Writing this book has been a process of integrating many areas of study and research under one umbrella. A common belief in naturopathic medicine is that everything is a process, and it is important to stay in the process and allow it to unfold; this book has followed that same belief. There have been many teachers, students, patients and friends that have assisted in the development of this book and I trust that many more will provide insight and information that will deepen and broaden the concepts that have been introduced.

There have been many people who have been instrumental throughout the development and writing of this book including: Dr Paul Saunders, Dr Dennis O'Hara, Dr Verna Hunt, Dr Pamela Snider, Dr Jared Zeff, Dr James Sensenig, Dr Christa Louise, Dr Mitchell Bebel Stargrove and Dr Jason Loken. I would also like to thank Nancy Bradley, Joy Gogh, Donna Seymour, Sher Smith, Dr Mary Jo Ruggeri and Dr Diane Manos who have been my teachers and supporters for many years. I am especially grateful to Dr Birgitta Jansen, Dr Carolyn Benson and Dr David Lescheid who graciously reviewed and provided endless support and feedback throughout this project. I would also like to thank my mother, Sherron Lloyd, and my partner, Hector D'Souza, who provide the foundation and support to allow me to live my dream and to work effortlessly.

SECTION I
PHILOSOPHIES AND SYSTEMS OF MEDICINE

CHAPTER 1
The changing perspectives of health and medicine from the ancient era to the postmodern era

The perspectives held about life, health, and disease have shaped and directed medical research, treatment options, public health policies, and the focus of health care and medical practices since the beginning of time. With every new discovery and invention, with changes in lifestyle and work habits, and as our environment and technology changes, medicine is impacted; sometimes for the better; sometimes for the worse.

The introduction of dissection, the understanding that disease can originate from external sources, and the continual discovery of new medical technologies contributed to our knowledge and understanding of health and disease. Even inventions such as gunpowder, the printing press, and plastics have played a role in shaping medicine. The ability to travel around the world transformed agricultural practices and has impacting medicine by adding a layer of complexity to disease etiology. The knowledge of the therapeutic properties of plants, chemicals, and minerals, and sound and light has shaped the treatment options available. Medicine and our understanding of life, health, and disease will continue to be shaped and transformed as the future emerges.

Different philosophies, models, and theories have accompanied the advancement of medicine; these have shaped the questions that were asked, the methods that were used to find the answers, and the way that the results were interpreted. Medicine has moved from theorizing about life based solely on the observation of nature, to researching the minute microscopic details of cells, to studying the intangible and energetic aspects of life. Our understanding of human beings is not yet complete, and being open to new ideas, and challenging the assumptions on which we base our current beliefs, is necessary to enhance our awareness of new possibilities and perspectives. The questions about life will always exist, and always change, as our insight deepens and new discoveries are made.

This chapter provides a brief look at the changing perspectives of health and medicine. It highlights factors that have impacted the development of medical systems, and that have influenced naturopathic medicine. Some of the beliefs and philosophies held in the ancient era, the Middle Ages, the Renaissance era, the modern era, and the postmodern era are explored. In many ways, the philosophies have come full circle. We once again believe that human life is integrated with nature (holism) and that there is a force, beyond ourselves, that guides us (vitalism). What has changed, is that we now have the research and ability to understand the concepts that before were taken on faith.

We don't have all the answers, but there is more of an acknowledgement that there are answers. The discussion of human life and medicine has been as much a philosophical discussion as it has been a scientific discussion. The time has come to see the value that all the pieces bring to our understanding of human life and the philosophy of medicine. Having an appreciation for the history of medicine is an important starting point in the understanding of how society views health, and why the practice of medicine is shaped the way it is.

Doc, I have an earache.

2000 BCE	*Here, eat this root.*
1000 BCE	*That root is heathen, say this prayer.*
1850 CE	*Prayer is superstition, drink this potion.*
1930 CE	*That potion is snake oil, swallow this pill.*
1970 CE	*That pill is ineffective, take this antibiotic.*
2000 CE	*That antibiotic is artificial, here, eat this root.*

Anon. History of Medicine

THE ANCIENT ERA

The earliest known civilizations lived in harmonious relationships with their surroundings. They held a holistic and vitalistic view of life and their explanations for life were based primarily on folk wisdom and subjective observation. Their pursuit of understanding the world and the human spirit were the same thing (Magner 1992). Linear causality and logical concepts were introduced in this era and the first dissections were performed.

The Eastern medical systems of Ayurvedic, Chinese and Greek–Unani medicine had existed for centuries and were based on holistic and vitalistic concepts. (These systems of medicine are expanded upon in Chapter 2.) Hippocrates (460–377 BCE) is considered the father of Western medicine. He based his views of health on the humoral theories of Greek–Unani medicine.

Health depends upon a state of equilibrium among the various internal factors which govern the operations of the body and the mind; the equilibrium in turn is reached only when man lives in harmony with his external environment (Foss & Borthnberg 1987).

Pythagoras of Samos (ca. 530 BCE), furthered this theory as he believed that the universe was composed of opposite qualities and the harmony, or balancing of pairs of qualities, such as hot and cold, moist and dry, was important in matters of health and disease. Alcmaeon, a pupil of Pythagoras, taught that health was a harmonious blending of each of the qualities with its appropriate opposite and that disease occurred due to excess or deficiency; for example an excess of heat causes fever, an excess of cold causes chills (Magner 1992).

Socrates (469–399 BC) used the term *logos* or 'will to live' to describe the vital principle present in man, yet the origins of vitalism are often associated with Aristotle (384–322 BCE). Aristotle developed a biological and materialistic approach to psychology where he believed that the 'soul' animated and directed the body. (González-Crussi 2007)

Much of the early understanding of how the inner body functioned was derived from dissections that were performed on animals, especially monkeys. Aristotle conducted dissections, yet most were not documented, and it is Galen (129–199 CE) who is credited with much of the initial understanding of anatomy as he performed and documented thousands of dissections.

Galen also introduced the concept that certain personality types were associated with particular diseases, and he reinforced the idea that the four elements of matter had 'qualities,' namely dryness, humidity, coldness, and heat. In his view, just as disease was thought to result from imbalances in the Hippocratic humors, it could also be caused by a number of factors that can disturb the respective qualities of these humors (Duffin 2007). After Galen, scientific knowledge was kept alive for years primarily by Arabic scholars who advanced the surgical art and study of internal medicine. They traveled extensively and established links with the traditions of the Far East, including India and China, and contributed greatly to the sharing of medical knowledge between these different cultures.

THE MIDDLE AGES

The European Middle Ages (500 to 1500 CE) was a period in which ideas about the nature of the universe, the nature of human beings, and their proper place in the universe – including their relationship to their Creator – underwent profound changes (Magner 1992). The Middle Ages saw the separation of medicine and surgery, the innovation of the hospital, and the challenge of devastating diseases. It was a period of transition from the Hippocratic traditions to medieval Christianity.

Ancient Greeks regarded good health as the highest good, yet seeking health was not congruent with Christian doctrine. According to Christianity, illness was regarded as a divine punishment for sins committed by the patient and healing required the spiritual and physical catharsis obtained by combining confession and exorcism with purgative drugs (Magner 1992). By the eleventh century, some monasteries were training their own physicians as it was felt that these physicians would uphold the Christianized idea of the healer who offered mercy and charity towards all patients, whatever their status and prognosis. Not everyone embraced these Christian concepts and hence the followers of Hippocratic medicine found ways to accommodate Christian beliefs and theologists found ways to justify the Hippocratic methods of healing.

The plague and leprosy contributed to the death of many and challenged the beliefs and ability of the current medical systems. The plague had been around previously but the outbreak in the fourteenth century was the most famous epidemic in Western history (Duffin 2007). The origins and transmission of disease, the concepts of resistance and immunity, and the necessity for proper hygiene were yet to be understood. This was a time of great learning as it contributed to the understanding of disease and the need for public health standards. For some, epidemics and disease were viewed as divine punishment, others felt they were brought by foreign travelers, and for most it was a time of great panic and suffering. Because of the inability of the church and their medics to handle diseases such as the plague, they lost a lot of credibility (Duffin 2007).

The Middle Ages was a difficult time for surgery and surgeons. Surgery was split into three classes. The highest class was the physicians who were university educated. Their role was to prescribe and to give advice. Next were hands-on practitioners who could dress wounds, set fractures, and apply poultices and plasters but who did not perform incisions or invasive procedures. Last were the 'barber-surgeons,' who were the 'untouchable caste,' so to speak, of the profession. They could bleed patients, lance boils, and perform other invasive procedures. They had no university education, and were regarded by their more exalted colleagues as menials (González-Crussi 2007). This distinction between the classes of medical men changed in 1540 when King Henry VIII signed a charter that incorporated barbers and surgeons in a common guild. Shortly after that medicine was established as a profession based on a formal education, standardized curriculum, licensing, and legal regulations.

Women have always been associated with the healing arts, yet from the twelfth century to the fourteenth century, although some Universities allowed women to study and teach medicine, women were discouraged or forbidden to practice formalized medicine. Hildegard of Bingen (1098–1179) was one of the twelfth century's most notable women (Magner 1992). She re-introduced the concept of treatments based on the principle of opposites and wrote about the medical uses and toxic properties of herbs, trees, mammals, reptiles, fishes, birds, minerals, gems, and metals. Other women served as nurses, herbalists, and healers.

THE RENAISSANCE ERA

Prior to the Renaissance (1300–1650), the philosophies held in the West were similar to those held in the East. In the West, the Renaissance period marked an artistic and intellectual awakening and a focus on objective measurements (Magner 1992). The body was starting to be explored using the concepts of chemistry and physics and the understanding of anatomy, physiology, and pathology were greatly enhanced. The Renaissance experienced a reawakening of the vitalistic concepts and an introduction of mechanistic concepts. This period saw the invention of the printing press, which resulted in the mass production of books, and the ability to compile and share information more easily. It also marked the time of increased travel and the introduction of new plants and remedies from foreign places. During the Renaissance, the focus of medicine was taken away from religious authorities and increasingly came more under the control of government and the state.

During this era there was a dramatic shift in how health and disease were viewed. The origin of disease was no longer viewed as a disturbance of the humors within the body, instead Paracelsus (1493–1541) postulated that there were disease-producing materials in food and drink. He also showed that disease was a chemical process that occurred locally in organs. This initiated the concept of abnormal organs as the primary seat of disease (González-Crussi 2007). Georg Ernst Stahl (1660–1734), a German physician and chemist, directed people's attention to the chemical processes of the human body, such as combustion, respiration, fermentation, and putrefaction. He believed that the soul regulated and harmonized the functions of the body, and that the body was subject to the laws of physics. 'He believed that since the soul governed the physiological phenomena, the conditions of the soul were the cause of health and illness' (González-Crussi 2007).

Significant medical discoveries changed the understanding of health and disease. For example, even though Chinese scholars had accepted the relationship between the heart, pulse, and the circulation of blood for centuries, William Harvey (1578–1657) is credited with discovering general circulation (González-Crussi 2007). This marked the mechanistic exploration of other bodily functions, such as digestion and metabolism. Many studies that followed were dismal failures because most of the chemical processes in the body were still unknown. In the eighteenth century, the relevance of chemical processes was confirmed when the French chemist Antoine Lavoisier demonstrated that respiration is a special form of oxidation (Capra 1996).

Human dissection had been part of the curriculum of some medical schools since about 1400, yet Andreas Vesalius (1514–1564) greatly enhanced the knowledge of anatomy as he did dissection on humans and worked with artists to create very high quality, detailed images of his dissections. Even still, it was not until the beginning of the nineteenth century, when the diagnostic techniques of percussion and auscultation made it possible to detect structural changes inside the chest, that anatomy became a major focus.

As a result of the new discoveries, naming of diseases with a precise diagnosis became important. This concept had been of little importance to the Hippocratic physician where the primary focus was the prognosis, which meant not only predicting the future course of the disease, but also providing a history of the illness (Magner 1992).

Names and concepts of diseases changed from being subjective symptoms, such as hemoptysis and shortness of breath, to associated anatomical lesions, such as pulmonary effusion, pulmonary consolidation, and emphysema (Duffin 2007).

THE MODERN ERA

The modern era (1650–1900) marked the emergence of scientific biomedicine. The philosophical and scientific foundations of this era were spear-headed by René Descartes (1596–1650) and Isaac Newton (1642–1727), and is marked by the concepts of reductionism, mechanism, and dualism. The underlying premise of this era was that the body and mind were viewed as separate from each other and separate from their environment and external factors. It was believed that diseases could be reduced to pathophysiological processes that could be understood solely based on a cellular and molecular level. Systematic, scientific study with randomized, double-blind control trials became the gold standard. This era contributed extensively to our understanding of disease, but it brought with it its own challenges.

The mechanists, influenced by Descartes' followers, 'widened the gap between science and spirit.' 'There is nothing included in the concept of the body that belongs to the mind,' Descartes said, 'and nothing in that of mind that belongs to the body' (Arntz et al 2005). Descartes initiated the concept of analytical thinking and his mechanistic approach shaped research and science for hundreds of years; it also contributed to man becoming more detached not only from his environment, but also from himself and his own mind and soul.

By viewing the world outside our minds as nothing but lifeless matter, operating according to predictable, mechanical laws and devoid of any spiritual or animate quality, it divided us from the living nature that sustains us. And it provided humanity with a perfect excuse to exploit all 'natural resources' for our own selfish and immediate purposes, with no concern for other living beings or for the future of the planet (Arntz et al 2005).

The ideas introduced by Descartes were enhanced by Newton, who developed a complete mathematical formulation of the mechanistic view of nature. (Capra 1996) In 1687 Newton wrote his treatise *Philosophiæ Naturalis Principia Mathematica*, which described universal gravitation and the three laws of motion that dominated the scientific view of the physical universe for the next three centuries. His work introduced the belief that the human body was a complex machine which could be reduced to the interaction of interchangeable physical parts. Two centuries later, Charles Darwin (1809–1882) supported the idea of separateness.

According to Charles Darwin life is random, predatory, purposeless and solitary...Life is not about sharing and interdependence. Life is about winning, getting there first. And if you do manage to survive, you are on your own at the top of the evolutionary tree (McTaggart 2002).

Darwin emphasized the idea that survival was about competition and strength; versus co-operation.

The knowledge gained of the inner workings of the body was immense. For example, the systematic work of Réaumur (1683–1757) addressed the question of how food and drink were broken down and absorbed into the body. It was recognized that there were certain organic entities, such as bacteria, that caused disease and that their effect could be avoided or reversed using certain substances (Foss & Borthnberg 1987). Also, in 1846 the use of anesthesia was discovered. As methods of controlling pain, hemorrhaging, and infection were discovered, the mindset and practice of surgery changed dramatically.

The modern era concepts were responsible for shifting the mindset of health care from that of preserving health, based on proper hygiene and lifestyle, to one of curing disease. Personal responsibility was no longer the focus; instead there was a belief that vaccines and drugs would treat any ailments that arose (Capra 1996). Medicine focused on what could be studied based on physiology and cellular pathology and, to a large extent, ignored the psychological and the psychosocial aspects. Biochemical processes were believed to function in a linear dimension of cause and effect. As new discoveries were made, such as the microscope, stethoscope, and X-rays, there became an even greater separation between the physician and the patient and between the patient and their symptoms.

There were great advances in science, but with that came even more unanswered questions. Immanuel Kant (1724–1804), a modern philosopher,

believed that science could offer only mechanical explanations, but he affirmed that in areas where such explanations were inadequate, scientific knowledge needed to be supplemented by considering nature as being purposeful (Capra 1996).

More challenges arose when the premises of biomedicine attempted to explain psychosocial factors in disease causation and when they attempted to explain many of the functions within the body. Théophile de Bordeu (1722–1776) proposed that there was a 'sensibility' that belonged to the material from which all living structures are made; as a vitalist concept, this 'sensibility' was not reducible to physiochemical terms (González-Crussi 2007).

The limitations of the reductionist model were shown as scientists tried to explain concepts such as cell development and differentiation, gravity, the ability of thoughts to influence functionality, and concepts of distant influences on cellular function. As science broadened, there were improved methods of researching the intangible and it became clear that there was more to the story.

THE POSTMODERN ERA

Early in the nineteenth century, revolutionary change started to take place, marking the start of the postmodern era. Quantum physics, thermodynamics, information theory, and the changes in the environment created paradigm shifts in the understanding of human beings, from a linear cause-and-effect biomedical model to a complex self-organizing biopsychosocial systems-focused paradigm. This era of complexity and diversity is characterized by the concepts of complex systems, holism, interactionism, and mutual causality.

In the postmodern era the term 'holistic' is used to mean two different things. First, it is a model in which the whole person – spiritual, mental, emotional, physical, social – is taken into account. Second, it refers to a model where the theoretical nature of the body posits a total interaction of all parts with each other so that none exists or functions independently. The 'holistic' model supposes a mutual causality relationship: the mind and body constitute an inseparable whole, where the whole is greater than the sum of its parts (Vickers 1998).

Systems thinking emerged simultaneously in several disciplines during the first half of the century, especially during the 1920s. The initial concepts were pioneered by biologists as a way of describing living organisms. It was further enriched by Gestalt psychology and the new discoveries in quantum physics.

In quantum mechanics a physical system is specified by a wave-equation that characterizes in one step both the material constitution of the system and its mode of operation – both its structure and its activity. There is no procedure for specifying that one independently of the other, and to speak of either in isolation is a mere abstraction (Toulmin 1967).

In the theory of irreversible thermodynamics, order emerges out of chaos and higher levels of organization out of lower orders (Prigogine 1978).

The most significant change in thinking involved the discovery that there was a field of light energy around all living things and seeing human beings as complex systems instead of machines. Machines function according to linear chains of cause and effect, and when they break down a single cause for the breakdown can usually be identified. Organisms are guided by cyclical patterns of information flow known as feedback loops. A multitude of interdependent factors are continually at play and which of the factors was the initial cause of the breakdown is often irrelevant (Capra 1988).

The postmodern era allows for the perceived contradiction between the modern era theories and the post-modern theories. Theories are valid for a certain range of phenomena, and traditional (modern era) assumptions are useful in many localized settings. The understanding of life itself is complex and cannot be broken down into a few limited theories or concepts. The post-modern era also recognizes that complete understanding is yet to be unraveled and might never be – human beings are dynamic complex beings of light energy. Chapter 4 explores some of the post-modern concepts in more detail.

REFERENCES

Arntz W, Chasse B, Vicente M 2005 What the Bleep Do We Know. Health Communications, Florida

Capra F 1988 The Turning Point, Science, Society, and the Rising Culture. Bantam Books, Toronto

Capra F 1996 The Web of Life. Anchor Books, New York

Duffin J 2007 History of Medicine, a Scandalously Short Introduction. University of Toronto Press, Toronto

Foss L, Borthnberg K 1987 The Second Medical Revolution. New Science Library, Massachusetts

González-Crussi FA 2007 Short History of Medicine. Random House, New York

Magner LN 1992 A History of Medicine. Marcel Dekker, New York

McTaggart L 2002 The Field, The Quest for the Secret Force of the Universe. HarperCollins, London

Prigogine I 1978 Time, structure and fluctuation. Science 201(4537):777–785

Toulmin S 1967 Neuroscience and Human Understanding. Rockefeller University Press, New York

Vickers A 1998 Examining Complementary Medicine. Stanley Thornes, Cheltenham

CHAPTER 2
Traditional and complementary systems of medicine

The traditional forms of medicine, such as Ayurvedic, Chinese, and Unani medicine, have been around for thousands of years. They are complete medical systems with an extensive history and philosophical understanding of the interrelationship amongst nature, life, health, and disease. Unlike Western medicine, they were not developed based on a scientific understanding of anatomy and pathology; instead they were based on observational qualities and characteristics of nature and human beings. The traditional forms of medicine have a set of principles that use a consistent language and are integrated throughout all components of the therapeutic encounter – the assessment, diagnosis, and treatment.

There are over 100 different complementary and alternative medical (CAM) practices that have developed over the last century. Some, like naturopathic, chiropractic, and osteopathic medicine, have clearly defined principles and philosophies and are systems of medicine that include assessment, diagnosis, and treatment. Other CAM practices have an auxiliary role and focus on a specific aspect of health or a single form of treatment. Most systems of medicine hold valuable information about the inner-workings of the human body and provide a 'piece of the puzzle' to our understanding of life.

> Every medicine is a language, a vocabulary of concepts that expresses fundamental beliefs about the nature of reality. It is through this grid that we perceive and explain ourselves (Beinfield & Korngold 1992).

The traditional medical systems of Ayurvedic, Chinese, and Unani medicine, as well as homeopathy embrace many of the same theories and principles of naturopathic medicine. As theories used in these traditional systems of medicine will be used to support the theories and concepts explored in this book, a short review of each of these systems is provided.

AYURVEDIC MEDICINE

History

Ayurveda is a holistic system of medicine that is indigenous to and widely practiced in India. The word Ayurveda is a Sanskrit term meaning 'science of life.' *Ayu* means 'life' or 'daily living' and *Veda* is 'knowing.' Ayurveda is a medical system that deals with health in all its aspects; physical health, mental balance, spiritual well-being, social welfare, environmental considerations, dietary and lifestyle habits, daily living trends, and seasonal variations in lifestyle, as well as treating and managing specific diseases (Pole 2006). Ayurvedic medicine was first practiced in India around 800 BCE. It has been influenced by the medical developments in the world, and has developed into a complete medical system with an extensive history and philosophical understanding of the interrelationship amongst life, health, and disease.

The basis of Ayurveda is that each individual has a unique constitution established at birth and influenced throughout one's life. How each person eats, lives, and interacts with their environment is based on this constitution. Ayurveda recognizes that seasons have a profound effect on health and that different seasons affect people differently. An individual's constitution and the seasons are intimately related. Health is affected by the qualities of the climate; the inner world is influenced by the outer environment (Pole 2006).

The five elements

Everything in life and nature can be explained according to the qualities of the five elements and these elements explain how the internal and external energies are linked together. Chapter 5 explores these elements in detail, but the following are some of the highlights (Svoboda 1988):

- *Earth* is a stable substance, the solid state of matter. It has the anthropomorphic attributes of stability, fixity, or rigidity.
- *Water* is a substance without stability. It is the liquid state of matter, whose attribute is flux.
- *Fire* is form without substance. Fire's characteristic attribute is transformation, as it has the power to convert a substance from solid to liquid to gas, and vice versa.
- *Air* is existence without form. It is the gaseous state of matter, whose attribute is mobility or dynamism.
- *Ether* has no physical form; it exists only as distances that separate matter in space and time. It is the field from which everything is manifested and into which everything returns; the space in which events occur.

The three humors (Doshas)

The five elements condense into three *doshas* – vata, pitta and kapha (Table 2.1). Each dosha has unique characteristics and determines a person's constitution. There are seven typical body constitutions based on the three doshas. Most people are a combination of the different doshas, but one dosha typically predominates. When the doshas are in harmony for an individual, a person will enjoy health; when there is disharmony, the functioning of the body is disrupted and leads to symptoms and disease.

The three doshas govern all the biological, psychological and pathophysiological functions of the body, mind, and consciousness. They act as the basic constituents and protective barriers for the body in its normal physiological condition; when out of balance, they contribute to disease processes. Each dosha has characteristic qualities, natural urges, preferences for food, temperature, and so on. They govern the creation, maintenance and destruction of body tissue, and the elimination of waste products from the body (Lad 1998). The doshas are described as follows (Svoboda 1988):

- *vata* is composed of ether and air. It is the principle of kinetic energy in the body. It controls movement throughout the body.
- *pitta* is composed of fire and water. It controls the body's balance of kinetic and potential energies. All of pitta's processes involve digestion or 'cooking,' even if it is the cooking of thoughts into theories in the mind.
- *kapha* is composed of water and earth. It is the principle of potential energy, which controls body stability and lubrication. The tissues and wastes of the body, around which vata moves, are kapha's territory.

Table 2.1   The doshas (Lloyd 2005, Burger 1998, Lad 1998, Svoboda 1998, Frawley 1989)

	Vata	*Pitta*	*Kapha*
Primary element	Air	Fire	Water
Secondary element	Ether	Water	Earth
Functions	Movement or propulsion	Transformation and conversion	Cooling and preservation
Characteristics	Stimulation, catabolic/ destruction, energetic humor	Growth, metabolic/ creator, thermogenic humor	Nurture, anabolic/ preservation, cohesive humor
Inner body functions	Movement and spaces in which the functions happen	Metabolism and secretions	Body structure and solidity
Digestive activity time	After complete digestion (elimination)	During digestion (enzymes and acids)	Start of eating (saliva and mucus)
'Seat' of expression	Colon	Stomach, Small intestine	Stomach, lungs
Subsidiary site	Nervous system	Gallbladder, bile	Lubrication, fat, plasma
Qualities	Dry, cold, light, irregular, mobile, rarefied, rough	Oily, hot, light, intense, fluid, malodorous, liquid	Oily, cold, heavy, stable, viscous, dense, smooth
Signs of excess	Dry or degenerative nature, underweight, interference with movement, cold, gas, constipation, restless worry, fear, anxiety	Heat or inflammation, bleeding, burning sensation, painful digestion, heartburn, yellow stools, anger, hypercritical	Overweight, increase in body mass or excess fluids such as tumors and swellings, mucus, heaviness, edema, nausea
Stages of life	55 years and older Metabolism slows down, tissues are not replenished as readily	Puberty to middle age Body needs to be maintained in stable state	Childhood Body grows – constant demand for nourishment to develop strong tissues
Time of day	2–6 (a.m. & p.m.) dawn/dusk	10–2 (a.m. & p.m.) midday/midnight	6–10 (a.m. & p.m.) early morning/ evening
Seasons	Fall/winter	Summer	Spring
Nature	Wind, oceans	Fire, sun	Rocks, mountains, moon, earth

The three gunas (Attributes)

Ayurveda encompasses the subtle attributes or qualities called *gunas* (Table 2.2). The doshas are a quantitative look at the qualities, the gunas are qualitative. The three gunas are sattva, rajas and tamas. 'These three attributes provide for the basis for distinctions in human temperament and individual differences in psychological and moral dispositions' (Lad 1998). All organic and inorganic substances, as well as all thoughts and actions, can be described based on these attributes.

Table 2.2 The gunas (attributes) (Lloyd 2005, Burger 1998, Lad 1998, Svoboda 1998, Frawley 1989)

Sattva	Rajas	Tamas
The cosmic force of equilibrium	The cosmic force of activity, motion or excitability	The cosmic force of inertia
Expression of essence, understanding, purity, clarity, compassion and love Normal, balanced state of a healthy mind	Mind operates on a sensual level, causes mind to be become overactive and unstable	Manifests in ignorance, inertia, heaviness, and dullness Excess causes the mind to become resistant to change
Subjective consciousness	Waves of kinetic energy	Material particles of potential energy
Spirit	Sense organs	Physical body
Ability to discriminate accurately	Excessive mental activity weakens discrimination	Insufficient mental activity weakens discrimination
Expression of essence, understanding, purity, clarity, compassion, and love	Mind operates on a sensual level	Manifests in ignorance, inertia, heaviness, and dullness
Comprehends well and follows their path steadily and consistently, progresses quickly	Full of hyperactivity, twist facts to fit their preconceptions, and convince themselves that they are progressing when they are in fact merely reinforcing external dependencies	Abundant inertia guides their being, they ignore clear evidence of the need to progress and dig in when they are in hope of remaining there
Promoted by healthful, simple, well-digested food and healthful, simple habits	Promoted by intense, stimulating foods and intense activities	Promoted by stale, putrid food and dulling activities (like too much sleep)
Promoted by milk, milk products, rice, wheat, mung beans, and most fruits and vegetables (avoid if allergic)	Promoted by salt, spices, sour foods, meat, fish, garlic, onions, and most legumes	Promoted by heavy, stale, indigestible foods and intoxicating substances
Associated with kindness, forgiveness, truthfulness, good memory, intelligence, ingenuity, courage, share joys and sorrows with others; not perturbed by good or bad, sorrow or joy, likes or dislikes	Associated with falsehood, cruelty, pride, boastfulness, sensuality, anger, cowardice, selfishness, afflicted with likes and dislikes too much, constant desire to be on the move	Associated with grief, unrighteousness, ignorance, foolishness, somnolence, avoidance of mental activity and physical work

The three malas

From the digestion of food and drink, the body produces the following three major waste products or *malas* – feces, urine, and sweat. The production and elimination of these is absolutely vital to health. According to Ayurveda, digestion is the most important function in the human body. The proper digestion, assimilation of nutrients, and the elimination of toxins is required to prevent disease. Ensuring that the body is able to properly eliminate all forms of malas is essential to Ayurvedic treatment (Srikantamurthy 1996).

Ama

The presence of *ama* in the body is considered the primary cause of disease. Ama is produced in the body as a result of improper digestion of food and drink. The presence of ama suppresses the enzymatic activity in the body, which is responsible for digestion, assimilation, and transportation of nutrients throughout the body and the functioning and production of tissues and organs.

> *Internal diseases begin with Ama, and external diseases produce Ama.*
> *In general, Ama can be detected by a coating on the tongue, turbid urine with foul odor, feces that contain undigested food or that have an offensive odor, and abundant gas. The principal course of treatment in Ayurveda involves the elimination of Ama and the restoration of the balance of the doshas (Micozzi 2001).*

Agni

Ayurveda medicine emphasizes the ability of the digestive fire to nourish the body and soul. The digestive fire is termed *agni* and it is seen as the metaphor for all metabolic functions in the body. It includes digestive function, sense perception, cellular metabolism, and mental assimilation. Agni is involved in many functions: absorption, assimilation, metabolism, digestion, perception, taste, touch, hearing, vitality, clarity, alertness, regular appetite, chemical combustion (Pole 2006).

Seven tissues

The chief functions of the body tissues are said to be, in order of importance: nourishing, enlivening, surrounding, lubricating, supporting, filling, and giving rise to an embryo (Frawley 1989). The tissues support and nourish the body and give it form.

Tissues have many vital functions, qualities, secondary tissues, wastes, and disease tendencies. Some theories of Ayurveda believe that there is a linear pattern: a step-by-step progression of nutrients transforming from one tissue type to the next. In this theory it means that a deficiency of plasma, for example, will lead to a deficiency of blood, which in turn will lead to a deficiency in muscle, followed by a deficiency in fat, etc. Another theory is that there is a progressive overflow of nutrients from one tissue channel to the next. In this theory the nutrients will 'feed' the reproductive tissue first, then the marrow and nerves, then bone, etc. A third theory is that each tissue takes the nutrients it wants from the central pool of nutrition, without the distribution being based on a hierarchical flow (Pole 2006).

The seven tissues are:

- *plasma* and skin contain nutrients from digested food and nourish all the tissues, organs, and systems
- *blood* governs oxygenation in all tissues and vital organs and maintains life
- *muscle* covers the delicate vital organs, performs the movements of the joints and maintains the physical strength of the body

- *fat* maintains the lubrication and oiliness of all the tissues
- *bone* gives support to the body structure
- *marrow and nerves* fill up the body spaces and carry motor and sensory impulses
- *reproductive tissue* contains the blueprint for all tissues, and is responsible for the development of life.

Ayurvedic assessment

The aim of Ayurvedic assessment and diagnosis is to identify the natural constitution of the patient, their mental status and the presence and severity of an abnormality. An assessment involves the site of origin of any disease, its path of transformation, and how it is being manifested in the body. Where a disease manifests in the body is often different from where it originated. For example, the disease might manifest in the digestive track, yet the cause originated due to a sense of disharmony in the mind.

An Ayurvedic practitioner will attempt to identify the causative factors (e.g. food, drink, mental state, lifestyle, seasonal influences) that resulted in the production of ama, and therefore the disruption in body functions, and the development of disease. An Ayurvedic assessment includes a history taking, visual observation, and physical exam that includes the examination of the radial pulses, body parts (tongue, skin, nails, physical features) and the analysis of urine. Diagnosis is communicated based on the qualities and characteristics of the doshas and the gunas.

Ayurvedic treatment

The aim of Ayurveda treatment is to establish a balance between the body humors. According to Ayurvedic teaching, the initiation of any form of treatment (whether it be herbal medication, acupuncture, chiropractic, massage, or any other) without first eliminating the toxins in the system that are responsible for the disease, will only push these poisons deeper into the tissues. Symptomatic relief of the disease process might result from superficial treatment. However, the fundamental cause of illness will not be affected and the problem will therefore manifest again in the same or another form (Lad 1998).

Ayurvedic treatment encompasses dietary guidelines based on the energetic qualities of food, gentle movement or yoga that is specific to an individual's constitution and disease state, specific daily routines including time of rising, sleeping, and bathing. It also includes massage, sweating, the prescribing of herbs and purification therapies (cleansing enemas, cleaning nasal medication, purgation, emesis, and therapeutic release of toxic blood).

CHINESE MEDICINE

History

Chinese medicine is a holistic system of medicine that has been part of the Chinese culture for over 3000 years. The ancient Chinese perceived human beings as a microcosm of the universe that surrounded them, and that they are motivated and driven by the same primeval forces of macrocosm. Optimizing human life by preserving the conditions within which it thrives is the purpose of Chinese medicine (Beinfield & Korngold 1991).

The philosophies and principles of Chinese medicine explain how the body works as an integrated system. The concepts of Chinese medicine closely parallel the theories that Western medicine is now discovering. For example, there is an understanding that the acupuncture meridians are channels of communication that follow the fascia; the systems theory supports the principle of the body as a networked system. Chinese medicine recognizes that the accumulation and balance of the attributes within an individual (Yin–Yang, heat–cold, blood–Qi) determines their internal climate, and therefore their health or disease.

Yin–Yang theory

Yin–Yang emerges out of oneness; this is the fundamental concept in Chinese medical philosophy. Yin–Yang represents complementary qualities that exist on a continuum; not opposite qualities. Nothing is purely Yin or Yang but a combination of them both. Yin–Yang is an expression of a duality in time, the fluidity of a continuum, and the cyclical movement of all of life. Everything can be explained based on the concepts of Yin–Yang (Maciocia 1998). This concept is explored in further detail in Chapter 5.

The human body is divided into Yin and Yang as follows: The internal region is Yin, whereas the external region is Yang; the five viscera are Yin, whereas the six bowels are Yang; and the tendons and bones are Yin, whereas the skin is Yang. In physiology, Yin stands for storage of energy, while Yang stands for human activities; Yin is held within the inner body to nourish the organs, while Yang stays in the superficial region to guard against foreign invasion (Kaptchuk 1983, Beinfield & Korngold 1991, Maciocia 1998). There is a constant interplay of Yin and Yang within and between all aspects of a human being.

Promoting a balance between Yin and Yang is a fundamental principle of clinical practice. The treatments based on this principle involve sedating the excess and toning up the deficiency. The Yellow Emperor's Classics of Internal Medicine states

> A hot disease should be treated by cold herbs; a cold disease should be treated by hot herbs... Yin should be treated in a Yang disease, Yang should be treated in a Yin disease (Lu 1994).

The five elements

The five elements are part of Chinese philosophy and refer to the nature of materials, as well as their interrelationships. The five elements differ from Ayurvedic elements and include wood, fire, earth, metal, and water. The five elements symbolize the direction of movement, the seasons, and all aspects of health and disease including physiology, pathology, diagnosis, and treatment. This five elements theory consists of four laws governing their relationships. These laws indicate how one organ can produce another organ,

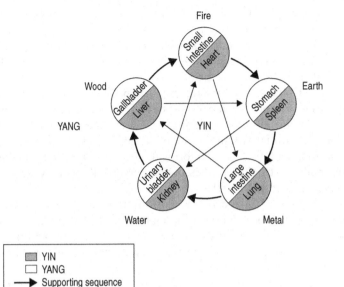

Fig 2.1 Five-phase organ network.

how organs control or attack each other, and how organs are able to resist control by another organ.

Each organ also has a literal and figurative function. For example, the spleen and stomach are responsible for the digestion and metabolism of food, as well as life. Every organ system is networked and linked to every other organ system and in every organ system there is a Yin organ and a Yang organ. Also, the internal aspects of all organs is Yin; the external Yang. The harmony between the organs is maintained by feedback loops that follow a specific sequence (Fig. 2.1). The supporting sequence represents the parent–child relationship between the organ systems, whereby one nourishes the next. In the restraining sequence one organ controls another ensuring that the balance within the network is maintained.

The vital substances

The body and mind are viewed as a complex network of energy and vital substances interacting with each other.

> *These substances manifest in varying degrees of 'substantiality', so that some of them are vary rarefied and some totally non-material. All together, they constitute the ancient Chinese view of the body–mind (Maciocia 1998).*

The vital substances are qi, essence, blood, and body fluids.

- *Qi* is the animating life force and substance. It is considered the essence of life and the origin of all other vital substances: thoughts and emotions, tissue and blood, inner life and outer expression (Beinfield & Korngold

1991). It is responsible for the generative and protective aspects of life. 'Qi is an energy which manifests simultaneously on the physical and spiritual level. It is in a constant state of flux and in varying degrees of aggregation. When Qi condenses, energy transforms and accumulates into physical shape' (Maciocia 1998).

- *Essence* in Chinese medicine refers to: prenatal essence, postnatal essence, and kidney essence. Prenatal essence is determined at conception and indicates a person's basic constitution. Postnatal essence is the energy that is received throughout life from food, fluid, and air. Kidney essence is the accumulation of them both, it forms the foundation for all functions in the body, and it naturally declines over a person's lifetime (Maciocia 1998, Beinfield & Korngold 1991).
- *Blood* is a form of Qi and is derived from the energy of food. Qi is the commander of blood; blood is the mother of Qi. The main function of blood is to nourish, maintain, and moisten the body (Kaptchuk 1983). From a Chinese point of view blood also carries the material foundation for the mind (Maciocia 1998).
- *Body fluids* originate from food and drink and refer to the water in the body. Their function is to lubricate internal organs, joints, muscles, skin, hair, membranes and cavities; and moisten and nourish the brain, marrow and bones (Lu 1994). Body fluids can be divided into clear fluids and turbid fluids. Clear fluids are spread throughout the muscles and membranes to moisten the muscles, skin, and hair, and they moisten the eyes, ears, mouth, and nose. Perspiration and urine are products of clear fluids. Turbid fluids are spread throughout the internal organs to nourish the brain, marrow, and bones and to lubricate the joints. They also nourish the muscles (Lu 1994).

Causes of disease

According to Chinese medicine philosophy, determining the cause of disharmony and disease is important in advising patients how to avoid, minimize, or prevent its occurrence. Chinese Medicine stresses balance as a key to health: balance between rest and exercise, balance in diet, balance in sexual activity, balance in climate, etc. Any long-term imbalance can become a cause of disease (Maciocia 1998). There are four main causes for disease:

- The *pathogenic factors* are wind, cold, summer heat, dampness, dryness, and fire. These factors are considered external if the attack is due to factors outside of the body, such as changes in climate during the four seasons. External factors attack the human body through the mouth, nose, or skin, and cause superficial diseases. Internal factors relate to conditions within the body, such as emotions, or the progression of disease.
- *Internal causes* typically refer to the emotions of joy, anger, worry, contemplation, sorrow, fear, and shock. These emotions can cause disease and, conversely, disorders of the internal organs can cause these emotions (Beinfield & Korngold 1991, Maciocia 1998).
- *Food* is essential to nourish the essence. From a Chinese medicine point of view, the energetic qualities of food, the regimen of eating, and the

balancing of food with seasons are all important. When food causes disease it is called a 'food injury'. Intoxification, overeating, eating greasy food, and eating food with cold or cool energies are common causes of 'food injury'.

- *Fatigue* is one of the factors that cause a deficiency state in the body. Fatigue might be of an internal organ or due to excessive sex. Fatigue due to an internal organ is a result of deficiencies in food or air; or due to excesses that have exhausted the body over time.

Chinese assessment and diagnosis

The aim of Chinese medicine assessment is to determine the qualities and characteristics of symptoms and disease. Detecting internal conditions through subtle external manifestations is the key to assessment in Chinese medicine. This is based upon the theory that any internal conditions will manifest externally. Thus, a physician is able to know about the internal conditions of a patient through such external manifestations as complexion, skin conditions, and verbal expression. The four methods of assessment are: observation, questioning the patient, hearing and smell, and taking the pulse. In clinical practice, the four methods are used in combinations (Lu 1994, Maciocia 1998). A Chinese medicine diagnosis is communicated based on the qualities of Yin–Yang and the causes of diseases.

Chinese medical treatments

The aim of Chinese medical treatment is to restore the Yin–Yang balance in the body. The treatments include: curing the spirit by living in harmony with the universe, dietary management, acupuncture, drugs (herbs), and treatment of the bowels and viscera, blood and breath.

> *In prescribing any preventive or therapeutic regimen, the physician had to carefully consider the influence of geography, climate, and local customs (Magner 1992).*

UNANI MEDICINE

History

Unaani means Greek and Unani medicine is an ancient Greek system of medicine based on the qualities of four temperaments and four humors. Unani medicine recognizes the mental, emotional, spiritual, and physical causes of illness or health and believes that each individual should take responsibility for their own well-being.

The threads that comprise Unani healing can be traced back to Claudius Galenus of Pergamum, who lived in the second century of the common era. The basic knowledge of Unani medicine as a healing system was collected by Hakin Ibn Sina (known as Avicenna) in 980 CE in Persia.

Subsequently, Ajmal Khan, who was born in India in 1864, is generally acknowledged to be the most significant twentieth century contributor to Unani medicine in India (Magner 1992).

Unani medicine, like Western medicine, originated with Hippocrates and his followers. The Unani system of medicine is practiced widely in Persia, Pakistan, and India. It is also practiced in South Africa, England and other countries. The Unani system is sometimes called Hikmat or Unani-Tibb.

Four elements

Unani medicine is based on the presence of the four elements fire, water, earth, and air. These elements are present in all aspects of life and in the body. Their balance leads to health and their imbalance leads to illness. The characteristic qualities of the four elements are similar to that of Ayurvedic medicine.

Four temperaments

The four temperaments are the foundational principle of Unani medicine. Everything in the universe – mineral, plant, animal, or man – consists of four elements and the qualities of heat, moistness, coldness, and dryness, in specific ratios. Depending on the ratios of these elements every object, compound or living entity has a state of equilibrium that reflects these qualities. The balance of qualities is called 'temperament' (Bhikha & Glynn 2007).

The four temperaments are classified as sanguinous (hot and moist), phlegmatic (cold and moist), bilious (hot and dry), and melancholic (cold and dry). Each individual and organ system will display a dominance of a specific temperament. The body fluids, also known as humors, are produced from food and drink, and are responsible for maintaining the balance of the temperaments. These humors are classified according to the same qualities.

Lifestyle factors

By choosing and regulating lifestyle factors health is maintained and disease can be prevented. The lifestyle factors recommend (Bhikha 2006):

- *Food and drink.* Regularly eating food and drinking enough water to sustain you in accordance with your temperament.
- *Environmental air and breathing.* Adjusting your lifestyle according to weather conditions, ensuring the air you inhale is clean, and that your lungs are working to full capacity.
- *Movement and rest.* Regular exercise suited to your temperament and pace of life, and ensuring enough leisure time and rest.
- *Sleep and wakefulness.* Getting the correct amount of undisturbed quality sleep, and feeling alert during waking hours.
- *Emotions and feelings.* Expressing and feeling emotions appropriately.
- *Elimination.* Effective elimination on a regular basis.

Unani assessment and diagnosis

The disorder of the humors is diagnosed through questioning, examination of pulse and tongue, and analyses of urine and stool. The communication of diagnosis is based on an individual's temperament and humors. Diseases, themselves, are also classified according to the temperament they manifest.

Unani treatments

All Unani treatments attempt to balance the four humors and assist the natural healing ability of the body. Addressing the lifestyle factors, including appropriate food preparation and selection, is an important first step to correcting an imbalance in the humors. If the condition is more advanced, a series of herbal formulations are used to 'ripen' and then 'purge' the offending humor (Bhikha 2006).

HOMEOPATHIC MEDICINE

History

Homeopathy was organized into a medical specialty by a German-born physician, Samuel Hahnemann (1755–1843) in 1807. The term *homeopathy* derives from the Greek *homoion pathos*, which means 'similar suffering'. By comparison, the term *allopathy* which refers to orthodox (conventional) medicine, comes from *allos*, meaning 'different'.

Hahnemann (1996) believed that there was a vital force within everyone that was responsible for health and healing. Homeopathy is based on the concept of holism and the belief that every part of the body is connected; physical symptoms elicit a psychological response, likewise psychological symptoms result in functional and structural changes in the body. To treat a complaint, therefore, it is necessary to treat the whole person, not just the part or organ that is affected.

The law of similars

Homeopathy recognizes that symptoms are a reflection of the body's attempt to heal, and hence remedies are chosen based on their similarity to the totality of symptoms – like cures like (Vithoulkas 1981).

> *Any substance capable of inducing specific signs or symptoms in a healthy person will be able, at low dosages, to alleviate these same signs and symptoms in a sick person suffering from them (Hahnemann 1996).*

The emphasis of the simillimum principle (treating like with like) is on enabling the patient's own self-regulatory and healing mechanisms rather than on manipulating and controlling body function and dysfunction (Swayne 1998).

Traditional and complementary systems of medicine

2

The 'totality of symptoms' principle

A classic homeopathic assessment involves a patient interview that initially takes 1–2 hours. The physician recognizes the uniqueness of each patient and looks at every part of the patient's life, from physical symptoms to preferences for foods and environment, to emotional temperament. The assessment includes a detailed history of how the symptoms developed, any concurrent symptoms, and how well the person actually feels at the time.

Illness always affects the whole person. Most physical symptoms elicit a psychological response; likewise psychological symptoms result in functional and structural changes in the body. In addition to the signs and symptoms of an illness, each patient will present their own unique signs and symptoms. Together, the unique signs and symptoms constitute the 'totality of symptoms' for each patient. The practice of homeopathy also recognizes that the manifestation of ailments differs considerably and these differences are important to consider. For example, some headaches come on suddenly, others gradually. Some headaches last very intensely for a short time, others are dull and can last for days, and some are intense for a long time. Choosing the correct remedy involves considering the patient's physical characteristics and temperament as well as the symptoms. A homeopathic assessment includes how the symptoms developed, any external factors, and how well the person actually feels at the time.

This attention to detail – the importance of taking seriously all that the patient has to say about the illness, and the belief that it all matters and has meaning – is a healing process in itself (Swayne 1998).

Homeopathic practitioners encourage patients to see themselves as an integrated whole, not as individual parts.

Homeopathic assessment and treatment

Symptoms are a reflection of the body's attempt to heal, and hence the aim of the homeopathic assessment process is to choose the correct remedy (simillium) that will address all levels of the individual and that will strengthen the body's defense mechanisms, assisting the body in overcoming an illness (Vithoulkas 1981). Homeopathic remedies are derived from plants, animals, and minerals. These substances are diluted, as the belief of homeopathy is that the smaller the dose, the greater the healing potential. Also remedies are selected on the basis of 'like cures like'.

Any substance capable of inducing specific signs or symptoms in a healthy person will be able, at low dosages, to alleviate these same signs and symptoms in a sick person suffering from them (Hahnemann 1996).

Dr. Constantine Hering, the father of American homeopathy, taught that the healing process progresses from the deepest part of the body to the extremities, from the emotional and mental to the physical, from the upper body parts (e.g. head, neck, ears, throat) to the lower body parts (e.g. fingers, abdomen, legs, feet). Hering's Law of Cure also states that healing progresses in reverse order and from the most recent condition to the oldest (Freeman 2001).

REFERENCES

Beinfield H, Korngold E 1991 Between Heaven and Earth, a guide to Chinese Medicine. Ballantine, New York

Bhikha R 2006 4 Temperaments, 6 Lifestyle Factors. Ibn Sina Institute of Tibb, South Africa

Bhikha R & Glynn JP 2007 Tibb: The Science of Medicine and the Art of Cure. Ibn Sina Institute of Tibb, South Africa

Burger B 1998 Esoteric Anatomy, the body as consciousness. North Atlantic Books, California

Frawley D 1989 Ayurvedic Healing, a comprehensive guide. Passage Press, Utah

Freeman L 2001 Mosby's Complementary & Alternative Medicine, a Research-Based Approach, 2nd edition. Mosby, Philadelphia

Frishman WH, Weintraub MI, Micozzi MS 2005 Complementary and Integrative Therapies for Cardiovascular Disease. Elsevier, St. Louis

Hahnemann S 1996 Organon of the Medical Art. Birdcage Books, Washington

Kaptchuk TJ 1983 The Web That Has No Weaver, Understanding Chinese Medicine. Congdon & Weed, Chicago

Lad V 1998 Ayurveda, the Science of Self-Healing. Motilal Banarsidass, Delhi

Lloyd IR 2005 Messages From the Body, a Guide to the Energetics of Health. Naturopathic Publications, Toronto

Lu H 1994 Chinese Natural Cures, Traditional Methods for Remedies and Preventions. Black Dog & Leventhal, New York

Maciocia G 1998 The Foundations of Chinese Medicine. Churchill Livingstone, Edinburgh

Magner LN 1992 A History of Medicine. Dekker, New York

Micozzi MS 2001 Fundamentals of Complementary and Alternative Medicine, 2nd edition. Churchill Livingstone, New York

Pole S 2006 Ayurvedic Medicine, the principles of traditional practice. Churchill Livingstone, Philadelphia

Srikantamurthy KR 1996 Clinical Methods in Ayurveda 2nd edition. Chaukhambha Orientalia, India

Svoboda R 1988 Prakruti, Your Ayurvedic Constitution. Geocom, New Mexico

Swayne J 1998 Homeopathic therapeutics: many dimensions – or meaningless diversity? In Vickers A 1998 Examining Complementary Medicine. Stanley Thornes, Cheltenham

Vithoulkas G 1981 The Science of Homeopathy. Grove Press, New York

Traditional and complementary systems of medicine

CHAPTER 3
Naturopathic medicine

HISTORY OF NATUROPATHIC MEDICINE

Naturopathic medicine, or naturopathy as it was first called, was established in America in the early twentieth century due to the efforts led by Benedict Lust. Initially, the practice of naturopathy included nature cure[1], homeopathy, spinal manipulation and other natural therapies (Kirchfeld & Boyle 1994). Like many of the founders of nature cure, Lust experienced the health benefits of this form of treatment first hand in an effort to overcome serious illness. Lust believed that the disease-oriented health care system of America was not working for many patients and he felt there was a need to get back to the roots of healing and to re-establish the link between health, disease, lifestyle, and the environment.

NATUROPATHIC MEDICAL PRINCIPLES AND PHILOSOPHY

Naturopathic medicine is derived from a strong philosophical belief about life, health, and disease. Its principles and philosophies are an integral component of naturopathic assessment, diagnosis, and treatment that represent a mind-set and approach for working with patients. Naturopathic medicine is more than just using natural agents and therapies for treatment. It is a model and set of operative principles and premises. It is this model, the approach to health and disease, the relationship that is established with the patient, and the focus on stimulating the natural healing ability of the body by identifying and addressing the disrupting factors, that distinguishes naturopathic medicine from other medical systems. The diagnostic and treatment processes are fundamentally patient-centered and health-focused; not disease or symptom focused. It is the assimilation of all the concepts that truly represents the naturopathic approach.

As primary care physicians, naturopathic doctors serve as a guide and an advisor to their patients. The process of healing involves addressing the link between life and health, and the importance of patient awareness and motivation. It is about recognizing the complexity and individualization of each patient and supporting the healing power of the body. Health and disease is a logical process; it happens for a reason. The aim of a naturopathic assessment is to find the reason(s), the root cause(s), and then develop an effective treatment strategy to address them.

The naturopathic principles and philosophy are:

- First, do no harm (*primum non nocere*)
- The healing power of Nature (*vis medicatrix naturae*)
- Identify and treat the root cause of disease. (*tolle causam*)
- Treat the whole person
- Disease prevention and health promotion.
- Doctor as teacher (*docere*)

---

[1]Nature cure is a term that refers to the use of natural agents, such as water, air, diet, herbs, and sunlight to treat disease.

First, do no harm (*primum non nocere*)

'First, do no harm' has been a principle of medicine since the time of Hippocrates and it refers not only to the patient but to the patient's vital force. It refers to choosing treatments that support the innate healing ability of the body and that honor the laws of nature. To 'do no harm', a practitioner chooses the therapy, and fashions the most gentle and non-invasive strategy to achieve the desired outcome for each individual patient. By respecting the integrity and vitality of the patient the healing process is supported versus overridden or suppressed. 'Do no harm' involves practitioners teaching their patients how to have more insight and awareness of how their lifestyle choices affect their health. It involves educating patients that more is not necessarily better.

When lifestyle factors are the root cause of disease or a contributing factor, it is important to address these factors in the initial part of treatment. Often when these factors are appropriately addressed, minimal or no other treatment is required; for example, a patient who has low energy due to poor dietary and sleep habits, or a patient who has stiffness due to being very sedentary and dehydrated. Ignoring the lifestyle factors negatively impacts the innate healing process of the body, and the patient's overall health. When supportive treatments are required they are chosen based on which treatments are the most gentle to achieve the desired outcome. In some situations, especially when the progression of disease is advanced or the current state of disease is critical, it is necessary to choose more aggressive treatments that have the potential for adverse effects. From a naturopathic perspective, there are no side-effects, there are only effects and these range from beneficial to adverse. Some adverse effects of drugs and other treatments occur when treatments are prescribed prior to, or in place of, addressing lifestyle factors, when a treatment is prescribed for longer than needed, or when an inappropriate treatment is prescribed for a patient. The aim of any treatment strategy is to minimize adverse effects.

'First, do no harm' is about choosing the most subtle and gentle treatment that establishes health or increases the patient's state of well being. It is not, as sometimes written, about only using gentle treatments. In some situations, for example, internal bleeding, fractures, or cancer, a radical approach is what is needed, but that does not mean it has to be invasive. It is possible to employ a potent approach, at the same time as supporting the healing power of the body. For example, a radical treatment strategy might mean a complete transformation of a person's lifestyle – such as, dietary changes, removing or addressing many external obstacles to healing at the same time, such as alcohol, smoking, recreational drugs, heavy metals, etc., increasing the amount of rest to allow for healing, spending time on a daily basis to actively address the psychological aspects of the illness, and taking time off work, changing one's daily lifestyle regimen and making substantial life changes. It might also involve naturopathic treatments, such as herbal medicines, supplements, homeopathy, acupuncture, physical alignment techniques or even treatments such as intravenous therapy to address and support the specific symptoms; or a radical treatment might involve the necessity for surgery or conventional medical intervention. The more any treatment is due to what the patient does (i.e. changes that they make) the more likely the healing.

Identifying and respecting the healing intention and capacity of the patient is an essential part of all therapeutic encounters. There is a difference between what is possible with supplements, drugs, and medication, and what is right to do. For example, in cases of palliative care, the patient might desire treatments aimed at improving quality of life, not necessarily at prolonging their life. There are a range of treatment intentions ranging from curative to balancing to supportive to managing to palliative to suppressive. At times, the patient's intention is limited due to their belief system or due to what they have read not due to the pathophysiology of their condition. For example, a patient who is diagnosed with fibromyalgia might read that there is no cure, and the only option that they have is to manage their pain. In situations like this, the practitioners might first re-educate the patient and provide the knowledge that when the disrupting factors which involve lifestyle, both environmental and psychological, are addressed there is the potential of a greater state of health than they currently anticipate.

The healing power of Nature (*vis medicatrix naturae*)

The healing power of Nature is an important principle of naturopathic medicine.

> *The basic philosophical premise of naturopathic medicine is that there is an inherent healing power in Nature and in every human being. It is the doctor's role to bring out or enhance this innate healing power within their patients (Pizzorno & Murray 1999).*

The definition of the healing power of Nature, according to the American Association of Naturopathic Physicians (1999), is 'the inherent self-organizing and healing process of living systems, which establishes, maintains and restores health.' This healing process is organized, ordered, and intelligent (Lipton 2005). It is the naturopathic doctor's role to support, facilitate and augment this process by identifying and removing obstacles to health and recovery, and by supporting the creation of a healthy internal and external environment. A naturopathic doctor Dr. Papadogianis wrote 'Within you lies a healing force more powerful than any treatment and more effective than any health-care practitioner' (Papadogianis 1998).

Throughout time, there have been many beliefs about disease and theories about healing. Hippocrates believed that everything in nature had a rational basis that followed the laws of Nature. The followers of Hippocrates used the term *vis medicatrix naturae*, the healing power of Nature, to denote the body's ability to heal itself (Murray & Pizzorno 1991). Georg Ernst Stahl (1660–1734) believed that the 'soul' was responsible for overseeing bodily functions and that the 'soul' held the power to heal.

> *Because there is a healing principle inside the body, the medical man is simply an assistant to Nature's curative potency, not a mechanic repairing a broken machine (González-Crussi 2007).*

Medical therapy can take two general forms: practitioners can attempt to strengthen the body so that it can heal, organize and defend itself, or they can attack the agents and mechanisms of disease directly. A naturopathic doctor addresses foreign agents of disease, but the focus is on strengthening the body thus decreasing its susceptibility to infection. When we cut our finger the body automatically knows what to do to stimulate the healing process and to close the wound. When we have the flu, the body initiates a fever and other efforts to kill the invading pathogens. When we eat spoiled food, the body responds by inducing vomiting or diarrhea. There is no mistaking that there is an innate healing ability to the body. The role of the doctor is to work with patients in order to identify the root cause(s) of disease and to remove the obstacles to cure. Naturopathic doctors support the creation of a healthy internal and external environment, they recommend that patients conserve vital energy and support the healing ability of the body, they work with patients to remove toxins, they assist in restoring structural integrity, and they encourage patients to adopt a healthy lifestyle.

Symptoms often are the manifestation of the organism's attempt to defend and heal itself.

The science of natural living and healing shows clearly that what we call disease is primarily nature's effort to eliminate morbid matter and to restore the normal functions of the body; that the processes of disease are just as orderly in their way as everything else in nature; that we must not check or suppress them, but co-operate with them (Lindlahr 1975).

For example, a patient complains of hip pain and numbness down his leg. If the patient has poor posture and continually sits on a thick wallet, the treatment involves correcting the misalignment, educating the patient on proper posture, and informing him not to sit on his wallet. When the flow of energy (or Qi), nutrients, blood, and nerve stimuli is returned to the area, the remaining symptoms often resolve on their own. Simply recommending an anti-inflammatory (whether drug, botanical, or homeopathic) does not address the root cause and even if the symptoms diminish temporarily, until the root cause is addressed, they likely will not completely resolve. The healing power of Nature is an innate process, but it is impacted by the choices that we make and the lifestyle and external factors that are imposed on the body.

Health is the natural state of the body. Maintaining health is the driving force of the innate healing response. When the optimal state of health is affected, the body aims to achieve the state of greatest health possible. The body compensates and diverts resources to ensure that life is sustained. According to Hering's Law of Cure, the body heals from the head down, from the inside out, and in the reverse order of the appearance of symptoms (Vithoulkas 1980). The body 'unwinds' as it heals, protecting the internal organs, thus providing the organs that are responsible for sustaining life with the resources they require. The more that the inherent healing ability and healing process of the body is supported versus overridden, the greater the depth of health achieved.

The healing power of Nature refers to both the body's innate ability to heal and the healing ability of Nature itself. The use of natural remedies has the power to stimulate healing. In fact, being in Nature itself can contribute to healing. This is discussed later in this chapter.

Identify and treat the root cause of disease (*tolle causam*)

We experience the body's ability to maintain homeodynamic functionality as health. When the homeodynamic functioning is overwhelmed, the body attempts to compensate. This compensation manifests as symptoms and as a disruption to health. The aim of the practitioner is to determine the specific trigger, signal, or patterns that initiated the disruption and that needs to be addressed.

Health and disease are complex and logical; the outcome of one versus the other occurs for specific reasons. The manifestation of disease is never the root cause of the problem. To understand the root cause a practitioner must start at when and why the disruption of health was initiated. To elicit a cure, the signal that initiated the imbalance – the root cause – needs to be addressed, especially if it is still signaling the body that there is a problem. For example, if a patient is angry because of the way they are being treated at work and they hold in their anger, this suppression of emotion might result in digestive discomfort, headaches, and red rash. If the treatment involves taking something to mask the digestive discomfort, medication for the headache, and a cream to minimize the redness of the rash, but does not address the anger, the suppressed anger continues to signal the body resulting in the same or deeper, more severe, symptoms.

Recognizing a relationship between lifestyle and health is a concept that has been around for centuries. In the 1600s, Thomas Sydenham, who is recognized as the founder of European clinical medicine, believed it was the task of the doctor to assist the body's natural processes while searching for the causes of disease (Magner 1992). Over the years, most people have moved further away from a lifestyle that is supportive of health. Fast food, stimulants, sedentary jobs, fast-paced lifestyles, and less time resting and sleeping are all contributing factors. The invention of pesticides, plastics, paints, cell phones, video games and more, have all had a negative impact on health. Human beings are complex, living, multi-dimensional energetic systems that have a limited capacity to handle the onslaught of a toxic lifestyle and environment. Identifying the root cause of disease and the aggravating factors is an essential aspect of health care. Nowadays there are just more factors. A practitioner needs to be more thorough with their history-taking and needs to recognize that there are contextual influences, external and environmental factors, and lifestyle factors that disrupt health and initiate signs of disease. As part of the therapeutic encounter, a naturopathic doctor needs to explore a much greater number of factors as health is improved by reducing the number of factors that strain the body and interfere with its normal functioning and ability to heal. Naturopathic treatment involves teaching patients that a return to a more simple and health promoting lifestyle often is the best medicine for them.

The body is complex and yet logical. It displays symptoms that correspond – provide a road map – to the root cause. For example, when a patient falls, their injuries correspond to how they fell and how they compensated. There are times when the physical manifestation of the symptoms and their corresponding root cause indicate a direct correlation and other times when the correlation is not as clear. Often when a patient is recalling their history they will use somatic metaphors to describe their symptoms or they intuitively link symptoms with events. For example, a patient recalls that their palms get sweaty and their heart races every time they have to speak to a certain person or speak in public. The primary issue that needs to be addressed is the anxiety associated with the event, not just the sweaty palms and the racing heart.

Identifying and treating the root cause of disease does not imply a linear causality between events in a person's life and disease. Human beings are a complex, dynamic and integrated system and it is the accumulation of multiple factors that contributes to health and disease. A specific event might be the primary trigger that initiated or amplified a series of symptoms, but their overall state of health, their adherence to lifestyle factors that are suited to their constitution, the impact of environmental factors, the support of family and community etc, all play a role in their ability to handle disrupting factors. The impact of any single event, at any point in time, depends on a number of other factors. The complex workings of the body follow the concept of mutual causality and recognize that the impact of any specific event is contextual and individual.

Treat the whole person (*tolle totum*)

Each patient's personal essence and the psychological, functional and structural aspects are an inseparable whole, that is, interconnected and interdependent with family, community and environment. The concept of a multi-dimensional individual differs significantly from the conventional model that generally focuses on the physical symptoms usually in isolation. 'Treat the whole person' is a holistic concept that recognizes that the whole is greater than the sum of the parts. There is also the recognition that each individual is unique with their own specific susceptibilities and way of manifesting disharmony and disease. The management of health and the progression of disease are complex processes that are influenced by many different factors. Naturopathic medicine recognizes that it is the harmonious functioning of all aspects of the individual, within the self and with their environment, that is essential to health.

Naturopathic medicine recognizes that each person has their own unique susceptibilities and ways of manifesting symptoms. This concept is shared in other medical systems. For example, according to Ayurvedic medicine, a person who has a vata constitution will be aggravated in the winter, with consumption of excess dry, cold food, by too much worrying, excessive movement, and if there isn't sufficient routine in their life. This is because vata relates to the qualities of cold and dry as well as to the mind and movement. For a person with this constitution when the season, their food and their lifestyle mirror these qualities versus balance them, they are more likely to be aggravated and hence symptoms relating to the aggravation appear (Lad 1998). Homeopathy is based on the understanding that the unique expression of an individual's symptoms is the most important criterion in the assessment process (Hahnemann 1996). For most traditional medical systems, and for naturopathic medicine, the concept of everyone having a unique makeup or constitution influences the assessment, diagnosis, and treatment of each patient. There is an understanding that you cannot separate the individual from their symptoms and the focus of treatment is to treat the patient, not the illness.

The principle 'treat the whole person' recognizes that human beings are complex and evolving systems. Understanding the complexity of individuals requires a practitioner to be able to look at a problem in all its dimensions. It requires the ability to synthesize (bring together), as well as the ability to analyze (to break things apart), and the recognition that living systems are dynamic, and non-linear.

> Changing one aspect of a system invariable changes all the others. Another important system's principle is that of hierarchy, every system is part of a suprasystem and it has one or more subsystems. A suprasystem of a human being would be the family. A subsystem of the human being would be the immune system. A subsystem of the immune system would be the lymph system, and the list goes on. ...No level excludes any other level, and all levels are equally important and work together (Louise 2007).

It also involves teaching patients to recognize the integration of all aspects of themselves and their surroundings. It is about encouraging patients to explore their life purpose, to be mindful of their habits and thought processes, to pay attention to their internal functions and posture, and to recognize the correlation between their life, their choices, and their health.

Disease prevention and optimal wellness

The *Huang Di Nei Jing*, a Chinese medical classic written in the second century BCE, states:

> Maintaining order rather than correcting disorder is the ultimate principle of wisdom. To cure disease after it has appeared is like digging a well when one already feels thirsty, or forging weapons after the war has already begun (Beinfield & Korngold 1991).

Preventive medicine involves assessing resources and risks and acknowledging how lifestyle and personal choices affect our health. Health and disease is, to a large part, a reflection of how an individual chooses to live.

Prevention of disease is a continual process that starts at conception and continues throughout all of life. It involves every aspect of a person's life, from their lifestyle, to their emotional health, the choices that they make, their family and community, and the environment that they live in. It is very difficult for individuals to be healthy, in an unhealthy environment. Individuals do have the ability to influence their lifestyle choices to a significant degree, for example, what they eat, their posture, their exercise and movement, and their daily regimen including sleep and relaxation. Symptoms indicate that something needs to change. The role of the practitioner is to facilitate increased awareness and to educate patients on the changes that are required, not only address these current concerns, but to ensure their prevention. Maintaining health and preventing disease is an ongoing process, not a short-term project.

Prevention of disease is a mind-set. It is about living a life of awareness, it is about self-responsibility and making choices conscious of their impact. It is about following the laws of nature, and implementing the principles of naturo-pathic medicine into daily life. Prevention of disease is a proactive approach to life and involves recognizing the interrelationship between individuals, their environment, their family and their community is an important aspect of this.

Health promotion and the degree to which a person feels well depends on their perception of wellness and often changes with different stages of one's life. According to Dr. William (Bill) Mitchell, a naturopathic doctor, 'body vital-ity + mental vitality + spiritual vitality = wellness' (Mitchell 2007). Body vitality includes the functioning of internal organs and systems, and a person's flexibil-ity, strength, and endurance and how strong and healthy a person physically feels. Mental vitality is a sense of well-being, feeling happy, experiencing and sharing love and thoughtfulness. Spiritual vitality is a sense of the greatness of the evolved universe, an appreciation of the efforts of people to understand the larger meaning of life and death, a humble and praisefull adoration of an omniscient guide (Mitchell 2007).

Wellness is a concept that many have attempted to define and measure. Some measurement scales include the spiritual, social, mental, emotional and physical. Others include concepts such as creative, coping, social, essential, and physical (Bell 2007). Some scales consist of solely one dimension, such as the physical, others emphasize the emotional. Wellness is an individual percep-tion; it changes with time and with the different experiences that one encoun-ters. It is the role of the naturopathic doctor to determine what wellness means to each patient and then to guide them in finding ways to achieve this.

Part of guiding a patient to wellness involves assessing risk factors and hereditary and lifestyle susceptibilities. It involves recommending appropriate interventions to prevent illness and taking steps to remove the obstacles to healthy function in order to stimulate the healing ability of the body. Other important factors affecting wellness include: intention, meaning, or purpose in life, one's perception of life and sense of hope. Having the intention to achieve wellness and believing that there is a purpose to life is necessary and valuable. Intentions refer not only to the patient but to the doctor as well. Inten-tion relates to the internal mind chatter, and the conscious and unconscious thoughts that a person has. If the thoughts are dysfunctional or doubtful of the ability to heal, they will adversely affect the healing process. It a person does not see the purpose to healing, if they have given up on life or feel that they would rather die, that too disrupts the healing process and the willingness that a patient has to comply with any treatment regimen or recommendation for lifestyle changes. Intention and purpose, on the part of both the practitioner and the patient, provide a focus, a direction and a guide in the therapeutic encounter and in the patient's healing journey. If a doctor recognizes that there is a concern at this level it is best addressed early in the treatment plan.

Doctor as teacher (*docere*)

Docere is the Latin word for 'teacher.' Teaching takes time and the therap-eutic encounter needs to allow sufficient time for the doctor to educate and teach the patient how to make and maintain the lifestyle choices and changes needed to assist them in achieving wellness. Many patients desire an under-standing of why they are sick, what they can do to improve the situation, and what they have to change for the future. It is this awareness and understanding by the patient that determines long-term wellness, not the knowledge level of the doctor. Thomas Edison wrote 'The doctor of the future will give no medicine, but will interest his patient in the care of the human frame, in diet and in the cause and prevention of disease.' 'The successful doctor of the future will have to fall in line with the procession and do more teaching than prescribing' (Lindlahr 1975).

There is nothing the Doctor can do...

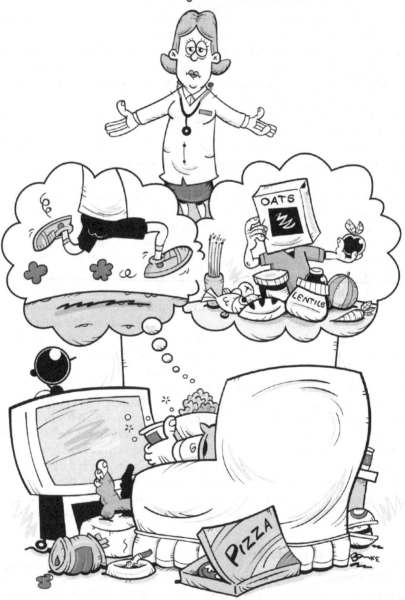

which will overcome what the patient will not.

With permission from the Canadian Association of Naturopathic Doctors.

The doctor is a facilitator and serves as a guide in the patient's healing process. It is the patient that does the healing; the doctor assists in the process. What the doctor brings to the relationship is the knowledge and the experience to appropriately guide the patient. The aim of the doctor is to establish a collaborative doctor–patient relationship, which in itself has inherent therapeutic value. By understanding the goals, healing intention, resources and limitations of the patient, the doctor can provide each patient with an individualized and evolving road map for their journey, and along the way they can educate patients and encourage self-responsibility for health. The greatest healing counsel a doctor can give to a patient is the knowledge and tools needed to establish and maintain their own health simply through living a healthy lifestyle that is in tune with their constitution and with nature.

NATUROPATHIC THERAPEUTICS

Naturopathic medicine has always encompassed a wide range of treatment approaches. These approaches are based on the principles described above and are often used concurrently in a treatment plan. The main therapies used by naturopathic doctors include:

- clinical nutrition
- botanical medicine
- homeopathic medicine
- Chinese medicine and acupuncture
- physical medicine including soft tissue work, therapeutic massage, naturopathic manipulation of muscle, bone or the spine, hydrotherapy techniques, gentle electrical impulses, ultrasound, diathermy, and exercise therapy
- prevention and lifestyle counseling
- psychological support
- intravenous and chelation therapy
- minor surgery
- colon therapy.

The scope of this book does not allow for a detailed breakdown of each therapy. There are many good books that provide this information.

NATUROPATHIC ASSESSMENT MODEL

Human beings are complex, dynamic systems with each part interacting and affecting every other part. Naturopathic medicine recognizes the interconnectedness of all aspects of a person, and that health is impacted by the individual's lifestyle and environment, as well as by external factors. Health is achieved by tuning the human body as a dynamic whole, not by addressing static individual parts. The optimizing of health is about facilitating a natural tendency towards alignment, coherence, and harmony among all aspects internally and externally.

The principles and philosophy form the foundation of naturopathic medicine. As naturopathic medicine evolves, the depth and wisdom of the principles takes on enhanced meaning and understanding. For example, research on complex systems supports the holistic view of an individual.

Quantum physics provides an explanatory mechanism for the ability of external factors to impact internal functions, for example, the ability of words to impact structure, and the ability of structural changes to impact function. Over the last couple of decades, many practitioners and scholars have looked at developing a more formal way of teaching the principles of naturopathic medicine. Figure 3.1 is a proposed model for naturopathic assessments. This model is based on the understanding that human beings are complex, dynamic systems; every aspect of the individual is interrelated, and human beings are a part of, and affected by, their environment. This model is depicted as two-dimensional, yet the concept is multi-dimensional.

Personal essence

The *personal essence* is a descriptive concept of an individual's vital or life force. Vital force is considered the primary force of all forces. It is the divine creative intelligence. The collective life force, or vital force, is a common pool of subtle energy that connects everyone together and interconnects people to their environment (McTaggart 2002). Personal essence refers to an individual's life force or vital energy, which comes from the collective life force,

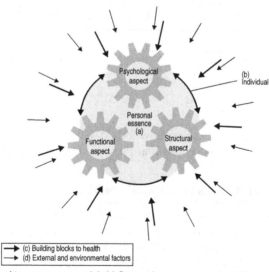

Fig 3.1 Naturopathic assessment model. (a) Personal essence – resides in the core and permeates every aspect of an individual. (b) Individual – consists of three distinct, yet interrelated components: the psychological, the functional and the structural. Each aspect is like a cogwheel that is able to influence every other component. (c) Building blocks to health – represents the lifestyle factors, essential elements, and behaviors that are needed to sustain life. (d) External and environmental factors – includes social factors, life experiences, environmental factors, medical interventions and all other external factors that impact health.

but is also individual and is, as such, impacted by personal factors. It recognizes the partial autonomy of the individual in the greater system of life.

The concept of 'vitalism', a subtle life force or essence guiding health and aiding in healing, dates back to the time of Hippocrates and Paracelsus (González-Crussi 2007). This concept is integral to Chinese, Ayurvedic, Unani, and homeopathic medicine, as well as other systems of medicine. According to homeopathy

> ...the material organism, thought of without the vital force, is capable of no sensation, no function, no self-preservation; it derives all sensation and performs all the functions of life solely by means of the immaterial being (the vital principle) which animates the material organism in health and in disease (Hahnemann 1996).

When the personal essence is strong and in harmony with the individual there is health. Imbalance, lack of harmony or coherence in the personal essence is a precursor (even an actual cause) of subsequent disease. The task of the individual is to learn how to live a life that is aligned with their personal essence and learn 'the language of the body' as it manifests signs and symptoms of imbalance indicating a need for change. The *Journal of Alternative and Complementary Medicine* declared that subtle energy or the invisible 'life force' is as much taken for granted as a fundamental fact of healing by alternative therapies as it is dismissed outright by the orthodox scientific medical world (Vickers 1998).

The personal essence resides in the inner core and permeates the psychological, the functional, and the structural aspects. It relates to our vital force, our sense of purpose, our spirituality and our connection with the collective consciousness. It provides a person with a sense of belonging to something that is greater than the self. The personal essence acts as a guide and a filter on a person's life. It holds a person's deep core beliefs and their values. It is their blueprint. This blueprint determines what they look like, their susceptibilities and influences, and how they perceive their world and interact within it. It determines an individual's sense of purpose and identity, and it impacts the pleasure and outlook that one has about one's life.

One aspect of the personal essence is a feeling of purpose; this purpose drives healing and provides the motivation on an ongoing basis to maintain a healthy lifestyle and to make healthy choices. As a guide and a filter, it determines the impact that situations and events have on a person's life. For example, a person may have worked hard to achieve a certain status or to acquire 'a good career' but once they have it they realize they aren't satisfied; there is an imbalance between their deep values and what they have. These deep values are held at the level of the personal essence. It is not a logical look at life, but that felt sense that says 'I'm on track; I'm doing what I was meant to do.'

The personal essence is impacted by the parents' health and their personal essence during conception. In Chinese medicine they speak of prenatal and postnatal essence. Prenatal essence is the energy that a child receives from their parents at conception; postnatal essence is the energy received from food, air, and water; together they determine a person's total essence. The personal essence is impacted, shaped, and developed throughout one's life, especially in the young developmental years. It is impacted by lifestyle choices. The personal essence needs to be 'fed' as much as the rest of the body. Many of the beliefs and values held in the personal essence are at an unconscious level, but they can be brought to consciousness through mindfulness, meditation, and other mental and spiritual exercises.

When an individual's personal essence strength is low or weak, it can impact their intention and desire to heal, and therefore their ability to heal. When the personal essence is the root cause of disease it is best to be addressed and acknowledged first. A person's personal essence has the ability to override the psychological aspect, to disrupt internal functions, and to impact a person's structure.

The aspects of an individual

An *individual* has three aspects – the *psychological*, *functional*, and *structural*. All aspects are inter-related; there is constant communication and feedback between and within each aspect. Each aspect is impacted by the tangible and intangible changes that continuously occur. To understand the communication and flow of energy from the psychological to the functional to the structural, it is helpful to see each as an expression of energy and each component as part of a complex system. For example, when an individual is under stress all aspects mirror and respond. There is a psychological impact such as impatience or irritability; the functional level responds with changes in breathing, heart rate, digestive capability, etc.; and there are structural changes, such as rounded shoulders or a collapsed posture. Each aspect of the individual carries the impact of the stress in its own way, and each conveys the same story.

The aspects of the individual are never the catalyst or cause of an imbalance or symptom. The individual simply displays the accumulation of the energetic wave patterns and the current homeodynamic state. For each human being there is a wave pattern that indicates health. When the wave pattern is in sync and in alignment, throughout the body, with the inner core and with the outer layers, we enjoy health. When there is misalignment or the waves are out of sync, we experience signs and symptoms of disease.

The psychological aspect

The *psychological* aspect relates to thoughts and emotions. It represents how we perceive ourselves and the world and how we communicate with our world and with ourselves. It is the sense we have of ourself in relationship to inner standards and external expectations. The psychological permeates the whole person and is able to influence all aspects of the individual.

The psychological is continually being shaped and influenced by our experiences, our environment and our state of health. There is an unconscious, conscious, and verbal or expressive aspect to the psychological component. The personal essence and the unconscious psychological aspect are closely related. The personal essence can be thought of as setting the unconscious expectations and the psychological as responding to the harmony between one's experiences and expectations. The unconscious holds the deep personal beliefs that influence our life, that responds to situations, and that 'filters' or assesses their impact and significance.

The conscious aspect of the psychological relates to the thoughts and emotions that we are aware of or that we can 'tune into' when we pay attention. It represents our ability to perceive and sense our bodily functions, to be aware of symptoms and our external environment. The verbal or expressive component of the psychological relates to how we communicate our thoughts, emotions, sensations, and perceptions. It is the exchange of our inner mental and emotional state with the outside world.

The psychological realm reflects the thoughts and emotions that someone has to their life and to their inner functionality and structure. At times the disharmony in the body is because of a lack of alignment between what we think or feel and what we express. When there is a lack of alignment, especially when it is chronic or when it is constant, it results in blockages in the flow of energy and hence in functional and structural changes. When an individual is overwhelmed, exhausted, or in a state of excess or deficiency, it impacts psychological responses, even to everyday events. Common examples of this are a person who becomes edgy when they are hypoglycemic (deficient), or someone who is agitated when they become hyperglycemic (excess). The functional state of the body often is a cause or an aggravating factor for psychological symptoms.

The recognition that the mind impacts health and disease is becoming much more understood. There are a vast number of areas of research looking at how the mind is able to impact health, for example, visualizations, biofeedback, positive affirmations, spirituality, prayer, and laughter.

The early pioneers in biofeedback and relaxation demonstrated that people could influence their own muscular reaction or heart rate, just by directing their attention to parts of it in sequence. Biofeedback even had measurable effects on brain wave activity, blood pressure and electrical activity on the skin (McTaggart 2002).

Even the placebo response, which can be considered a psychological belief, results in physiological changes. The placebo effect is an important part of the healing process. Another profound aspect of the psychological in respect to the healing ability of the body is intention.

Intention is the midwife of actualization, and if the intention is to heal and become well, then there is a much greater likelihood of that occurring than if the patient is hopeless and without intention of becoming well (Mitchell 2007).

Different emotions have different qualities and hence different impacts on health.

Destructive emotional vibrations obstruct the inflow and normal distribution of the life forces through the organism, while the constructive emotions of faith, hope, cheerfulness, happiness, love and altruism exert a relaxing, harmonizing and vitalizing influence upon the tissues of the body (Lindlahr 1975).

Naturopathic medicine

43

The observation that emotions relate to organs and that they reside in different parts of the body is fundamental to both Chinese and Ayurvedic medicine. Later in this book the properties of individual emotions and thoughts are explored.

The impact of specific events or situations depends on the strength and resilience of the psychological aspect of the individual. For example, the feeling of fear accompanies a situation that threatens a person's sense of wellbeing. The degree of fear is a reflection of the threat that is perceived. If there is an underlying sense of a lack of safety the person's reaction might seem, to others, more extreme than the situation warrants. If, on the other hand, the reaction to the same threat is characterized as a calm reaction, we would expect to find a stronger sense of inner safety. An individual's psychological response is based on their constitution, and the accumulation of experiences, and it will either mirror or complement the situation that they are currently faced with.

Assessing the psychological state is accomplished primarily in the holistic intake. As a practitioner masters the ability to listen to a patient's story, to hear the somatic metaphors in what a patient says, to question in a way that allows a patient to peel the layers to reveal the patterns and to uncover the root cause(s) of disease, the impact of the psychological aspect is revealed. The role of the practitioner is to determine whether psychological factors are stimulating healing or inhibiting healing; whether it is reflecting a cause of disease, mirroring the impact of the disease or a result of some other imbalance in the individual.

The functional aspect

The functional aspect relates to the inner organs, glands, tissues and body fluids. It relates to how the body systems interact and communicate at the system, organ, and molecular levels. It involves the movement of fluid and energy between the cells, and within the cells, tissues, and organs. Both the psychological and structural aspects are able to override and influence its ability to operate; it is also able to override theirs.

The functional body has been the primary focus of conventional medicine for centuries as it has been the most easily analyzed and studied. Tools such as laboratory testing, radiographs, magnetic resonance imaging scans, and ultrasounds give practitioners an important perspective on what is happening at a cellular, organ system, and physiological level. The functional assessment reveals the current state of health and the progression of disease. It provides insight into the aspects of the body that are manifesting the disharmony, how the body is compensating, and the progression of disease

The functional aspect is the 'work-horse' of the body. It relates to the systems such as the immune, respiratory, cardiovascular, digestive, musculoskeletal, endocrine, or nervous. Each system has organs, tissues, and body fluids that have an optimal range that must be maintained and preserved in order to sustain their role, function, and existence. Every part of the inner body adapts and compensates in order to maintain its role, each component is part of the whole and influenced by every other aspect. The preservation of each part is done by the body's innate intelligence and its self-sustaining and self-regulatory ability. When the body is in a state of 'overwhelm', either due to excesses or deficiencies, the role of an individual might be modified or sacrificed in order to sustain life of the whole. For example, if an individual is in a deficiency state, it is common for the blood flow in the periphery to be sacrificed (decreased) to ensure that the internal organs can still function.

The functional body is responsible for assimilating and absorbing the nutrients and elements from the external environment. It is the functional body that links each person to Nature. The self-sustaining and healing ability of the body requires nutrients, water, and air. The air we breathe, the food we eat, the water we drink, are all processed by the body. Ideally, the body breaks down and absorbs what it needs and eliminates what it doesn't need. The ability of the body to excrete toxins is an essential aspect of health. If the organs of elimination are blocked, or aren't working efficiently, it impacts health. The main organs of elimination include the lungs, skin, bowels, and kidneys. Routes of elimination also include menstruation and the expression of ideas and emotions. In naturopathic medicine, a major aspect of the treatment plan is to ensure that the organs are functioning and efficiently eliminating toxins and waste.

The structural aspect

The structural aspect represents the physical matter, the form, shape, outline, and alignment of the physical body. It relates to the physical structure of a person – the somatic body or the outer body – and to the structure and form of organs and tissues. It represents the tangible aspects of an individual. The structural aspect is the most crystallized manifestation of an individual's energetic constituents.

A person's structure provides the foundation and the container for the body. It protects and supports a person literally and figuratively. When aligned, it allows for organs to function appropriately, bodily fluids to flow unimpeded, and for harmonious energetic cellular communication; structure governs function. When there is misalignment or imbalance, it results in functional and psychological changes in the body. A person's structure is affected by many different factors, such as, posture, gait, ergonomics, excesses or deficiencies in movement and exercise, nutritional level, lifestyle and even a person's clothing and shoes. It is impacted by a person's constitution, their occupation, their muscle strength and the frequency and amount of load that they carry.

The conventional approach to structural analysis is to look at muscles, ligaments, cartilages, bone, etc in a fairly mechanical way, with the emphasis being on the structure of the individual parts. 'Diagnosis is only a matter of applying one's anatomy' (Magee 1997). From a holistic and naturopathic perspective, the focus includes the function of each structural part and its relationship to the rest of the body. Symptoms of structural imbalance often indicate or include local and distal structural concerns. For example, neck pain can be caused by misalignment of the back, hips, knees, and even the feet.

There are serious limitations to the conventional medical approach. The most serious is the tendency to focus on the site of the symptoms and to ignore the context, which is the whole organism – the person. Because the structures are emphasized, there is a tendency to look for and to treat structural changes in the affected tissues and to ignore important general factors such as constitution, general health, nature of work and psychological factors. (Legge 1997)

Assessing the structural systems involves observation and palpation. Often, areas of misalignment are visible simply by observing how a patient sits, stands, or moves. During a patient history, as a patient becomes more comfortable with the practitioner, or as they become more guarded, it is important to observe structural changes. A patient's structure changes as they discuss different events in their life, especially if the events are still impacting them. For example, if a patient is talking about an embarrassing situation it is typical for their posture, especially their chest, to collapse. It is important to maintain a holistic approach when assessing structural or musculoskeletal complaints.

The assessment of structural complaints is reviewed in Chapter 9.

Building blocks to health

The building blocks to health represent the human factor in health and disease. They are the essential elements and the lifestyle factors that provide the nutrients and 'fuel' to sustain life, to move, and to function. Naturopathic medicine believes that both the quality and the quantity of the building blocks to health are important. The significance of any one is unique and depends on a patient's constitution. The building blocks are the foundation of disease prevention and health promotion. They influence all stages of life and all stages of health and disease. There is ample research to support their importance in disease prevention and their role in chronic disease, yet they are often overlooked or minimized as part of a conventional medical assessment and treatment strategy. The building blocks include:

- conscious breathing
- proper nutrition/dietary regimen
- adequate clean water
- proper posture and physical alignment
- fresh air and sunlight
- exercise/movement
- sleep/rest
- expression of emotions/thoughts
- healthy mental outlook and mind chatter.

Historically, health and disease have always been linked to lifestyle factors. During the modern era, medicine started to pull away from the relationship between lifestyle and health and doctors began to treat the body as a machine, separate from its environment. As we enter the post-modern era, there is a return to the realization that humans are connected to their environment, that lifestyle is a key determinant of health, and that life and health need to be thought of, assessed, and treated as one.

The average westerner has an unhealthy, disease-promoting lifestyle, but the tools that a typical medical doctor has (i.e. drugs and surgery) never address this underlying factor. Although effective when appropriately applied (such as surgery for appendicitis), drugs and surgery often have too many side effects to be used in the treatment of many early, common and/or recurring problems people have (Murray & Pizzorno 1991).

Even the decline in infectious diseases began with addressing hygiene and sanitation. The maintenance to these factors continues to be an integral part of the health for the world's population. To a large degree, especially in developed nations, the building blocks to health are under an individual's direct influence, or under the influence of an individual's care-giver. Human beings are able to make choices and decide the degree to which they choose health as a way of life. Unfortunately, for many people, convenience, external factors, and short-term desires tend to win over personal long-term health and wellness. The result is that health is getting worse and chronic illnesses and lifestyle diseases, such as diabetes, high cholesterol, and heart disease, are on the rise. What is even more disconcerting is that the conventional treatment approach is based on the same principles that caused the problem – that is short-term outcomes versus long-term health. From a naturopathic perspective, the approach to lifestyle diseases and chronic illness starts with self-responsibility and decisions based on the long-term health of not only the individual, but the environment in which they live.

The building blocks are a way to prevent disease and they are the way to address chronic illness and lifestyle diseases. They can be the root cause of disease when they are in excess or deficiency for any length of time, or when they are misaligned with an individual's life and constitution. When the building blocks to health are the cause of a patient's health concerns, the impact is usually gradual. The body has internal reserves and when they become depleted or exhausted, a patient's strength and resilience declines. Even when the building blocks are not the root cause, they often are an aggravating factor and an obstacle to cure, and need to be addressed as part of a naturopathic treatment. Implementing the building blocks to health is about ensuring that the daily regimen is based on healthy choices, and are based on what a patient needs at any given point and time depending on the stage of disease, seasons, current stressors, etc.

The way and degree to which a patient incorporates the building blocks into their life influences their vitality and ability of the body to heal, grow and repair. The body is self-sustaining and self-regulating; it continuously repairs and heals to the best of its ability. When the body is in a state of disease, there might be a need for a patient to decrease the time they spend involved in 'external' endeavors and increase their focus and attention to the building blocks of health and to personal rejuvenation. The following highlights the importance of the specific building blocks to health.

Breathing is one of the most important physiological functions of the body. Taking a breath signals the start of life, and taking your last breath signals the end of life. Breathing has a voluntary control as well as a reflex control. It directly affects the nervous and circulatory system, the lungs, and the mind. It is closely linked to the psychological component and is the first of the physiological functions to change in response to changes in emotions or thoughts. Breathing fulfills three key objectives: respiration and gas exchange, acid–base balance, and communication. Breathing is also instrumental in assisting an individual becoming focused and grounded.

The brain cells begin to die after just four minutes of oxygen deprivation, therefore the body will sacrifice anything to make sure we keep breathing. For example, people develop forward head posture within 5 minutes of a respiratory obstruction, and because of the 'survival reflex', if respiration is dysfunctional any treatment for a musculoskeletal disorder is only palliative and temporary. Optimal breathing function is linked to most functions in the body and improper breathing or decreased lung capacity is associated with many diseases.

Food provides the human body with nutrients. The act of eating, and the nutrients in what we eat nourish the body, mind, and soul. Food allows the body to grow and develop, it also is used to prevent and cure disease (Lu 2000). The nurturing effect of food depends on the quality and quantity of food, as well as the eating regimen and the environment in which one eats.

Nutrition is generally regarded as a twentieth-century science, yet the belief that health and long life depend on the regulation of food and drink is an ancient and universal principle of medical theory. Classifying food from the perspective of its constituents, such as protein, carbohydrates and fats and vitamins and minerals began in the nineteenth and twentieth centuries and it is helpful when we are looking at mapping the molecular and chemical composition of the body.

Quite simply, (a healthy diet) is a diet which provides optimum levels of all known nutrients and low levels of food components which are detrimental to health, such as sugar, saturated fats, cholesterol, salt and additives (Murray & Pizzorno 1991).

The energetic properties contribute greatly to the understanding of how to utilize food to maintain health for different constitutions and how to restore balance within the body. Food is classified in terms of opposing qualities such as hot or cold, light or heavy, moist or dry. These qualities determine the impact of food internally and whether a particular food is strengthening, weakening, purgative, or constipating. Foods can also be classified according to their flavors, such as pungent, sweet, sour, bitter, or salty. Eating according to the energetics of food is used to balance constitutional tendencies and in times of illness to balance the disharmony in the body. For example, if an individual is always cold, eating cold food might intensify the problem; while eating food that warms the body and food that is cooked versus raw helps with balancing the cold (Svoboda 1989).

Water is one of the most common and essential components in the body. It is responsible for many vital functions including cellular communication and the transport of all bodily fluids. It is a life-sustaining and life-giving substance that is required for every living function, including the elimination of waste products. Without sufficient water on a regular basis the body soon becomes dehydrated. A lack of water affects energy, health, and longevity.

Posture represents the ability of the body to maintain structure and form. An aligned posture provides open pathways for the flow of bodily fluids and energy. An individual's constitution dictates what 'normal' posture is, recognizing that normal is not always straight and symmetrical. Posture is affected by everything that an individual does, by emotions, exercise, and ergonomics, how a person walks and stands, whether they have a tendency to cross their legs or fold their arms, etc. For example,

> some habitual posture changes might place a greater strain on the
> musculoskeletal system, computer use by adolescents should be viewed as
> a possible health concern (Straker et al 2007).

Addressing postural concerns or modifying posture is beneficial in the treatment of many health concerns, for example,

> sitting upright or in a semi-sitting position reduces venous return in patients
> with heart failure, intracranial pressure in patients with intracranial
> hypertension, intraocular pressure in glaucoma patients and may decrease
> the gastro-oesophageal reflux (Martin-Du Pan et al 2004).

Fresh air and sunlight are essential to the survival of all living things and spending time outside, breathing fresh air, and being around nature is beneficial to health. Interaction with nature reduces depression, promotes healing, sparks creativity, and even increases life expectancy-upping survival odds by about 15% over 5 years (Mahoney 2007). Being in Nature is reported to make people feel more grounded, more connected to Nature, and to have a better sense of purpose and direction (Lyndon 2002). Most people know that they feel better when they are outside, yet an increasing number of children, and adults, are spending more time inside. Not only are they not enjoying and utilizing the health benefits of being outside; they are also usually more sedentary and glued to a television or computer.

Noise pollution, light pollution, or living in man-made environments such as cities with wall-to-wall concrete and asphalt is disruptive to health. Overall, the quality of air is a major world-wide problem and a growing public health concern (Bartra et al 2007). Many of the impurities in the air, the toxins and the pollutants are invisible to the human eye, but have the ability to cause both acute and chronic effects on human health, affecting a number of different systems and organs. The impact ranges from allergies to minor upper respiratory irritation to chronic respiratory and heart disease, lung cancer, acute respiratory infections in children and chronic bronchitis in adults, aggravating preexisting heart and lung disease, or asthmatic attacks. In addition, short- and long-term exposures have also been linked with premature mortality and reduced life expectancy (Bartra et al 2007, Kampa & Castanas 2008).

Movement is the body's ability to flow in space. On the structural level it represents the flexibility and strength of the body. On a cellular level, it relates to cellular communication and the transfer and movement of bodily fluids. External movement is required to aid and support the internal flow of bodily fluids. For example, walking supports the movement of blood and lymphatic fluid back to the heart; deep abdominal breathing is needed for the diaphragm to 'massage' the liver and maintain the position of the stomach (Klotter 2003, Lane et al 2005). The internal movement of energy often is mirrored externally; internal congestion or disruption results in external constriction and decreased range of movement.

Every component of the body has an optimal range within which it functions. For example each joint has its own range-of-motion, the movement of the eyes is designed to optimize peripheral vision and expansion of the lungs is greater with deep abdominal breathing versus shallow chest breathing. Every part of the body needs to be used, strengthened, and reinforced with the awareness of the impact, on an ongoing basis in order to maintain optimal movement.

Regular exercise or movement is beneficial as it enhances the transport of oxygen and nutrients to the cells and the transport of waste products from the body. It improves cardiovascular and respiratory function and maintains the tone, flexibility, and strength of muscles and joints.

Regular exercise not only makes people look better, but also makes them feel better. Tension, depressions, feelings of inadequacy and worries diminish greatly with regular exercise (Murray & Pizzorno 1991).

Rest and sleep represent the body's ability to slow down, to heal, to turn inward, and to grow. It is reflected by the central nervous system being in a parasympathetic mode versus a sympathetic mode. Sleep disorders might be primary, or more commonly, a secondary symptom of the advancing disease process (Hajjar 2008). In acute situations, insomnia and restlessness often are due to an overactive mind, physical pain, itchiness, consuming too many stimulants such as caffeine, inadequate darkness, or feeling of uneasiness within oneself (Omvik et al 2007, Roehrs & Roth 2008). Every aspect of the body needs to rest. The mind needs to be able to shut off to allow for a deep sleep. Digestion and other internal functions work best when they have periods of rest, and muscles need to recover after exercise. Quiet time, mindfulness exercises or meditation all assist an individual in slowing down and provide time for the mind to reflect, integrate information and to appreciate their life.

Expression of emotions is essential to health. It is one of the secondary emunctories, or routes of eliminating toxins; such as toxic thoughts or feelings. When a patient experiences strong emotion, it is important that they have an outlet for expression. The outlet can be verbal, written, or through bodily expression, such as exercise or gardening. What is important is that a patient acknowledges their emotions, understands the root cause, and has ways of expressing them. When there is a difference between what is felt and what is expressed it creates a sense of disharmony and lack of coherence or alignment within the body. This disharmony contributes to disease. For example, a woman is unhappy with her marriage, her job, and her life, and she feels sad and 'depressed'. This sadness is a true reflection of her life. Recommending a treatment that suppresses her sadness, without her making any life changes intensifies the disharmony. What she requires is either to 'reset' her expectations or, as is often the case, to make changes in one or more aspects of her life.

The *mind* relates to a person's thoughts, both conscious, and unconscious. As psychological aspects of an individual, the mind and emotions can alter the functional and the structural aspects. The mind can stimulate the healing process, intensify the impact of subtle interventions, or it can nullify the impact of an extensive treatment intervention. A person's mind chatter, mental state, expression of thoughts and emotions, and their outlook on life are all important contributors to health.

Environmental and external factors

The number of external factors and the degree of their impact is increasing all the time. The more awareness that an individual has about the health impact of the external factors they encounter, the more options that they have to lessen their impact. Environmental and external factors need to be included as part of every assessment. The following is a list of common external factors grouped according to five main categories: life events, social factors, environmental factors, external factors and medical factors.

Life events refers to the experiences that we have throughout our life. It represents the situations and events that have had an impact, both beneficial and adverse. It refers to any accidents or injuries that we have had, the subsequent treatment, and result of those treatment(s). Life events relates to the choices that we make such as choosing to smoke, to take recreational drugs, or to consume alcohol and it includes exposures during prenatal development.

Every experience in our life impacts our health. The body is an accumulation of it all. Personal growth and health is affected by how we perceive the events and situations that we encounter. We can learn as much, or more, from adversity as we can from prosperity. Events that we view as beneficial add to our sense of confidence, our belief in ourselves, our sense of strength and personal ability. Experiences that provide exposure to new places and situations allow for a greater appreciation of ourselves, for a deeper awareness of individual differences, and an understanding of how human beings fit into the greater scheme of things. When we see life events realistically and we appreciate the learning that they provide, we end up with greater resilience and a more vital personal essence.

When an individual is faced with a difficult situation, the body initially goes into stress mode as it processes the situation. For example, when you are fired from a job, someone close to you dies, or you are in an accident, the stress response heightens. At the same time, the inherent healing processes are initiated. Physically, the body starts the repair process; psychologically, it starts to process and determine the next steps and the impact of the situation. On every level, an individual works to restore a new homeodynamic state. If, for any reason, the healing is blocked, then the situation continues to affect health. For example, it is common and natural for someone to grieve the death of someone they love. If, 10 years later they are still in a state of grief then their health is still being affected. If you are fired from a job and 2 years later you are in a new job and 'have gotten over' being fired than the situation no longer is sending signals of disharmony. If, on the other hand, you have a new job and you are still angry that you were fired, it is still affecting you. As a patient recalls the significant events in their life what you, as the doctor, are listening for is situations where the patient is still emotionally 'triggered'. Any situation that still has a negative impact on a patient is detrimental to health; situations that have a positive impact strengthen health.

Social factors refer to the people in our lives who affect us. It relates to our family, community, and work environment. Family can have a beneficial or adverse impact on a person's health; it all depends on the history and dynamics. For many people, their primary social support comes from their family; also the ability to love someone and feel loved is important to health. Family is responsible for much of a person's learned behavior, their belief systems, their coping skills, their communication skills, and their attention to and focuses on health.

Community for some is their immediate environment; for others it represents a cultural, age or religious group and for some it represents professional or business affiliates. Community is our wider support network. Usually there is a common belief system, a common focus or interest. Research shows a correlation with increased health, the feeling of being part of a community and the creation of health promoting settings (Masotti et al 2006).

Environment encompasses many different factors and has a tremendous impact on health. The seasons, for example, have always contributed to the psychological sense of well-being. Many people feel better simply because the sun is shining. People tend to be more active in the summer. The winter time, with the decrease in sunlight, often has been associated with lower mood states, increased melatonin levels, and increased demands for nutrients, such as vitamin D (Morera & Abreu 2006).

Over-population and industrial technology have contributed in various ways to a severe degradation of the natural environment upon which we are completely dependent for life (Capra 1982). The environment also impacts health and disease because of the presence and exposure to toxins, heavy metals and chemicals. There is an increased concern about the prevalence of toxins in food, soil, water, and air. Health hazards caused by heavy metals have become a great concern to the population. Lead, mercury, arsenic, and cadmium are the most important current global environmental toxicants. These heavy metals affect the functioning systems, including the central nervous system, circulatory, reproductive and urinary systems, producing serious disorders (Sattler 2005, Flora et al 2007, de Burbure et al 2006). Screening for heavy metal accumulation is becoming a necessary part of treatment, especially for chronic diseases. The number of deleterious chemicals that we are exposed to increases all the time. There is increasing knowledge about the impact of chemicals on health and the need to decrease the amount of chemicals being used in food, storage containers, cooking utensils, household products, etc.

External factors are increasing all the time. The chemicals in personal care products, additives in foods, plastics bottles, fillers, and metals used in dental procedures, heavy metals, the quality of water and air, the impact of pesticides, fertilizers; the list goes on and on. Each one impacts specific biological processes, inhibits the proper absorption or distribution of nutrients, and often contributes to disease. Heavy metals, for example, include both those essential for normal biological functioning (e.g. Cu and Zn), and non-essential metals (e.g. Cd, Hg, and Pb). Both essential and non-essential metals can be present at concentrations that disturb normal biological functions, and which evoke cellular stress responses. The organs and systems most commonly affected by heavy metals include the kidney, liver, heart, and the immune and nervous systems. Decreasing the concentration of heavy metals in the body therapeutic effects on certain diseases (Lynes et al 2007).

Medical factors include all forms of treatment that a patient has undergone, such as surgery, chemotherapy, radiation, reconstructive surgery, and any drugs and supplements that a patient takes. Some medical interventions, such as surgery, are necessary to sustain life or to address serious or life-threatening disease states. From a naturopathic perspective, what is important is the intention and reasoning for the treatment, whether the root cause for the illness was ever addressed, and how the innate healing ability of the body has been impacted. The assessment of medical interventions involves addressing the implications of drugs and nutrients and the impact of medical treatments and procedures. It is important to recognize the difference between supporting the healing ability of the body and overriding the wisdom of the body. Drugs, and nutrients to some degree, often are prescribed without the root cause being addressed. Often they are prescribed based on symptomology and are only addressing the symptoms, instead of addressing the cause, or addressing the pattern of disharmony. The short-term and linear thinking of prescribing is dangerous to health and contributes to the progression of disease. For example, although drugs for blood sugar regulation might result in decreasing fasting blood sugar levels, they do not slow down the progression of diabetes, and might contribute to the early onset of diabetic complications.

There are many unintended reactions to medications. As part of any assessment it is important to investigate the medications that patients are taking, their adverse effects and interactions, their contraindications, and their routes of elimination. Understanding the current health status of a patient, while on medications, involves addressing the impact of the medications on health and recognizing that the normal innate reactions and self-regulatory functions of the body do not operate the same when a patient is medicated.

REFERENCES

AANP, 1999 www.AANP.org American Association of Naturopathic Physicians

Bell I 2007 A Multivariate Empirical Approach to Modeling the Vital Force. Foundations of Naturopathic Medicine Project, Washington

Beinfield H, Korngold E 1991 Between Heaven and Earth, a Guide to Chinese Medicine. Ballantine Wellspring, New York

Capra F 1982 The Turning Point, Science, Society, and the Rising Culture. Bantam Books, Toronto

de Burbure C, Buchet JP, Leroyer A, et al 2006 Renal and neurologic effects of cadmium, lead, mercury, and arsenic in children: Evidence of early effects and multiple interactions at environmental exposure levels. Environm Health Perspect 114(4):584–590

Flora SJ, Flora G, Saxena G, Mishra M 2007 Arsenic and lead induced free radical generation and their reversibility following chelation. Cell Molec Biol 53(1):26–47

González-Crussi FA 2007 A Short History of Medicine. Random House, New York

Hahnemann S 1996 Organon of Medicine, sixth edition. B Jain Publishers, New Delhi

Hajjar RR 2008 Sleep disturbance in palliative care. Clin Geriatr Med 24(1): 83–91

Kampa M, Castanas E 2008 Human health effects of air pollution. Environment Pollut 151:362–367

Kirchfeld F, Boyle W 1994 Nature Doctors, Pioneers in Naturopathic Medicine. Medicina Biologica, Oregon

Klotter J 2003 Lymphatic System & Exercise. Townsend Letter for Doctors & Patients 238:p26

Lad V 1998 Ayurveda The Science of Self-Healing. Motilal Banarsidass, Delhi

Lane K, Worsley D, McKenzie D 2005 Exercise and the lymphatic systems: implications for breast-cancer survivors. Sports Med 35(6):461–471.

Legge D 1997 Close to the Bone, The Treatment of Musculo-Skeletal Disorder with Acupuncture and Other Traditional Chinese Medicine, second edition. Sydney College Press, Australia

Lindlahr H 1975 Philosophy of Natural Therapeutics. CW Daniel, England

Lipton B 2005 The Biology of Belief, Unleashing the Power of Consciousness, Matter & Miracles. Elite Books, California

Lousie C 2007 Systems Principles and Naturopathic Philosophy: The Human Being as a Complex System. Foundations of Naturopathic Medicine Project, Washington

Lu HC 2000 Chinese System Foods for Health and Healing. Sterling Publishing, New York

Lyndon A 2002 Get Outside, Get Happy. Natural Health 32(8):90–96

Magee DJ 1997 Orthopedic Physical Assessment, third edition. WB Saunders, Philadelphia

Magner LN 1992 A History of Medicine. Marcel Dekker, New York

Mahoney S 2007 The Fresh-Air Fix. Prevention 59(8):193–195

Masotti PJ, Fick R, Johnson-Masotti A, Macleod S 2006 Healthy naturally occurring retirement communities: a low-cost approach to facilitating healthy aging. Am J Public Health 96(7): 1164–1170

McTaggart L 2002 The Field, the Quest for the Secret Force of the Universe. HarperCollins, Great Britian

Mitchell B 2007 The Vis Part 1 and 2. Foundations of Naturopathic Medicine Project, Washington

Morera AL, Abreu P 2006 Seasonality of psychopathology and circannual melatonin rhythm, J Pineal Res 41(3): 279–283

Murray MT, Pizzorno JE 1991 Encyclopedia of Natural Medicine. Prima Publishing, California

Omvik S, Pallesen S, Bjorvatn B, Thayer J, Nordhus IH 2007 Night-time thoughts in high and low worriers: reactions to caffeine-induced sleeplessness. Behavioural Research Therapy 45(4): 715–727.

Papadogianis P 1998 Treat the Cause, Naturopathic Solutions for Common Health Concerns. Prentice Hall, Scarborough

Roehrs T, Roth T 2008 Caffeine: Sleep and daytime sleepiness. Sleep Med Rev 12(2):153–162

Sattler B 2005 The risky business of reproduction: environmental exposures and associated risks to fertility and healthy babies. Zero to Three 26(2): 20–25

Straker LM, O'Sullivan PB, Smith A, Perry M 2007 Computer use and habitual spinal posture in Australian adolescents. Public Health Reports 122(5):632–643

Svoboda RE 1989 Prakruit, your Ayurvedic constitution. Geocom, New Mexico

Vickers A 1998 Examining Complementary Medicine. Stanley Thornes, Cheltenham

Vithoulkas G 1980 The Science of Homeopathy. Grove Press, New York

FURTHER READING

Alricsson M, Landstad BJ, Romild U, Gundersen KT 2008 Physical activity, health, BMI and body complaints in high school students. Minerva Pediatr 60(1):19–25

Bartra J, Mullol J del Cuvillo A, et al Air pollution and allergens. J Investig Allergol Clin Immunol 17(2):3–8

Bonefeld-Jørgensen EC, Long M, Hofmeister MV, Vinggaard AM 2007

Endocrine-disrupting potential of bisphenol A, bisphenol A dimethacrylate, 4-n-nonylphenol, and 4-n-octylphenol in vitro: new data and a brief review. Environm Health Perspect 115(1):69–76

Calafat AM, Ye X, Wong LY, Reidy JA, Needham LL 2008 Exposure of the US population to bisphenol A and 4-tertiary-octylphenol:2003–2004. Environm Health Perspect 116(1):39–44

CAND, (2005) www.CAND.ca Canadian Association of Naturopathic Doctors

Cohen M 2007 'Detox':science or sales pitch? Austr Fam Physic 36(12): 1009–1010

Davies D, James TG 1930 An investigation into the gastric secretion of a hundred persons over the age of sixty. BMJ 1–14 In Murray M, Pizzorno J 1991 Encyclopedia of Natural Medicine. Prima Publishing, California

Djeridane J, Touitou Y, de Seze R 2008 Influence of electromagnetic fields emitted by GSM-900 cellular telephones on the circadian patterns of gonadal, adrenal and pituitary hormones in men. Radiat Res 169(3):337–343

Dossey L 1985 Space, Time & Medicine. New Science Library, Boston

Dworak M, Schierl T, Bruns T, Strüder HK 2007 Impact of singular excessive computer game and television exposure on sleep patterns and memory performance of school-aged children. Pediatrics 120(5):978–985

Grof S 1990 The Holographic Mind. Harper, California

Hardell L, Sage C 2008 Biological effects from electromagnetic field exposure and public exposure standards. Biomed Pharmacother 62(2):104–109

Hulme C, Long AF 2005 Energy healing training and heart rate variability. J Altern Complement Med 11(3): 391–395

Jansson M, Linton SJ 2006 The development of insomnia within the first year: A focus on worry. Br J Health Psychol 11(3): 501–511

Koezuka N, Koo M, Allison KR, et al 2006 The relationship between sedentary activities and physical inactivity among adolescents: results from the Canadian Community Health Survey. J Adolesc Health 39(4):515–522

Kordas K, Lönnerdal B, Stoltzfus RJ 2007 Interactions between nutrition and environmental exposures: effects on health outcomes in women and children. J Nutr 137(12):2794–2797

Krupp MA, Chatton MJ 1984 Current medical diagnosis and treatment. Lange Medical Publishing, California In Murray M, Pizzorno J 1991 Encyclopedia of Natural Medicine. Prima Publishing

Martin M 2004 Naturopathic Philosophy: Time is of the Essence. Journal of the Australian Traditional-Medicine Society 10(2)

Mellman TA 2006 Sleep and anxiety disorders. Psychiatr Clin N Am 29(4):1047–1058

Myers S 2007 Whole Person Medicine. Foundations of Naturopathic Medicine Project, Washington

Pizzorno JE, Murrary MA 1988 A Textbook of Natural Medicine. John Bastyr College Publications, Seattle

Pizzorno J, Murray M 1999 Textbook of Natural Medicine, second edition. Harcourt Publishers, Seattle

Rey-López JP, Vincente-Rodríguez G, Biosca M, Moreno LA 2008 Sedentary behaviour and obesity development in children and adolescents. Nutr Metab Cardiovasc Dis 18(3):242–251

Roth T 2007 Treatment and management of chronic insomnia. Primary Psychiatry 14(5):1–10

Roth T, Krystal AD, Lieberman JA III 2007 Long-term issues in the treatment of sleep disorders. Int J Neuropsychiatr Med 12(7):10:1–15.

Shilo L, Sabbath H, Habari R, et al 2002 The effects of coffee consumption on sleep and melatonin secretion. Sleep Med 3(3):271–273

Stargrove MB 2007 A Cosmology: Context for the Process of Healing. Foundations of Naturopathic Medicine Project, Washington

Tarhini AA, Kirkwood JM, Tawbi H, et al 2008 Safety and efficacy of arsenic trioxide for patients with advanced metastatic melanoma. Cancer 112 (5):1131–1138

Turner RN 2000 Naturopathic Medicine, Treating the Whole Person. The principles and practice of Naturopathy. Thorsons, UK

Vogel A 1959 The Nature Doctor. Bioforce-Verlag Teufen, Switzerland

Walverkar RR et al 2007 Chronic arsenic poisoning: a global health issue – a report of multiple primary cancers. J Cutan Pathol 34:203–206

Wasserman GA et al 2008 Developmental impacts of heavy metals and undernutrition. Basic Clin Pharmacol Toxicol 102(2):212–217

Whitelaw G 1998 Body Learning, How the Mind Learns from the Body: a Practical Approach. A Perige Book, New York

Wood C 1998 Subtle energy and the vital force in complementary medicine. In Vickers A 1998 Examining Complementary Medicine. Stanley Thornes, Cheltenham

Zeff JL 1997 The process of healing: a unifying theory of naturopathic medicine. J Naturopath Med 7(1):122

SECTION II
THEORIES, PATTERNS AND DEFINITIONS OF HEALTH AND DISEASE

CHAPTER 4
Human beings as complex, dynamic systems of energy

Historically, much of the conventional medical research and meaning of health was determined by what the physical body was doing on a chemical and structural level. There was the recognition that thoughts and language play a role in disease, but the interpretation, all too often, started and ended with cellular processes. Human beings were viewed using mechanistic and dualistic concepts; they were treated as separate from their external environment, and the mind was viewed as separate from the body.

These old beliefs were challenged for years as there were many unanswered questions. For example, the speed of communication could not be explained by the key and lock analogy that was used to explain communication across cellular membranes. There was no clear explanation of how the body was able to handle multiple tasks simultaneously, how language, thoughts, and emotions elicited specific physiological changes, or how the environment or social factors impacted health. There was also little knowledge of how memory was stored or retrieved or what initiated or controlled functions such as growth, development, or longevity (McTaggart 2002).

The perception and understanding of how human beings function and survive has been broadened and continues to expand based on new discoveries. Systems theory supports the concepts of vitalism and holism and provides a framework for explaining the complexity and dynamic interconnectedness of all aspects of life (Capra 1996). The discovery that electrical fields of energy are the foundation of life provides increased knowledge about cellular communication and how endogenous and exogenous factors affect health (McTaggart 2002). Together, these theories provide a model that supports the principles used in the naturopathic assessment of symptoms and diseases.

This chapter explores human beings as complex, dynamic systems of energy. The aim is to provide a sense of the complexity and intrinsic nature of human beings, an appreciation for the organizational structure, and the relationships that exist. What becomes evident is that one aspect cannot be separated from another, and to assess health and disease you have to understand the tangible and the intangible aspects of human beings, the environment that they live in, the universe at large, and the interplay that occurs as things interact and change.

WAVES OF LIGHT ENERGY

The fundamental basis of life is electrical fields of energy. Everything in the world, regardless of how dense it is, or whether it is tangible or intangible, is composed of electric charges that interact with other energetic fields (Haisch et al 1994, Hunt 1996). Human beings are not simply biochemical beings, but energetic and informational beings that interact and communicate on a constant basis both within themselves and with their external world (Oschman 2003).

The presence of electrical fields around living things was first studied in the 1940s by Harold S. Burr, a neuroanatomist from Yale University (Burr 1972). He discovered that all sorts of organisms, from molds, to salamanders and frogs, to humans, possess an electrical field. He also discovered that the electrical fields change with stages of growth, seasons, sleep versus waking, and between health and disease (McTaggart 2002).

In the 1970s and 1980s the researcher Fritz-Albert Popp was studying the effects of electromagnetic radiation on living systems. What he revealed was that all living things – from the most basic of plants or animals, to human beings – emitted a permanent current of photons and that these vibrations of light are a major component of the communication system of the body (Oschman 2003). What he also discovered was that the number of photons that an organism emits is linked to their position on the evolutionary scale and to their degree of health. The more complex and healthy an organism, the fewer photons they emit. Hence, rudimentary animals and plants have a very high frequency of electromagnetic wave, within the visible light range, whereas humans emit much far photons (Popp et al 1992, Hunt 1996).

Both the tangible and the intangible possess an electrical field that emits light. The frequency of electrical fields that correspond to the biochemical and biological processes in the body, are detectable as frequencies that belong to one or more radiation bands in the electromagnetic spectrum (Sylver 2008). The electromagnetic spectrum represents the different energy 'oscillations' and wave patterns that comprise our known universe (Fig. 4.1). It ranges from the slower-moving, lower-energy electrons of electrical current to the faster-moving, higher energy photons of visible light and other wavelengths.

The different fields of light energy interact and are linked by electromagnetic energy. This interlinking creates a coalesced wave form that holds the properties and qualities of each component and has its own unique vibrating light energy. This ability of waves to interact, to store and carry information is the means of cell-to-cell communication and occurs in response to internal and external signals (McTaggart 2002, Oschman 2003).

Human beings emit a coalesced light vibration that represents the whole person, and an individual light vibration for each organ system, down to a specific light vibration for each individual cell, tissue, molecule and atom. The interaction and coalescing of the energetic fields of light establishes the foundation for life and for bodily functions. In essence, human beings are simply a networked collection of energy that functions as a unit within a larger sphere of energy.

The more a wave pattern manifests as a tangible structure the more slowly it changes; the more intangible, the more quickly it changes. For example, thoughts and moods are intangible and can change very quickly; organs and tissues are tangible, they continually change and regenerate, but more slowly – sometimes to the point of looking fixed in their structure. Because wave patterns hold the accumulation of all the information that they have encountered, they provide the body with the ability to remember how to look and act, to remember past events, and to remember how to perform different tasks (McTaggart 2002). Wave patterns provide a much more complete explanation of how the body is able to manage multiple, complicated tasks in different parts of the body instantaneously.

All wave patterns have a characteristic frequency, amplitude, wavelength, and phase (Fig. 4.2) (Sylver 2008). As wave patterns encounter each other

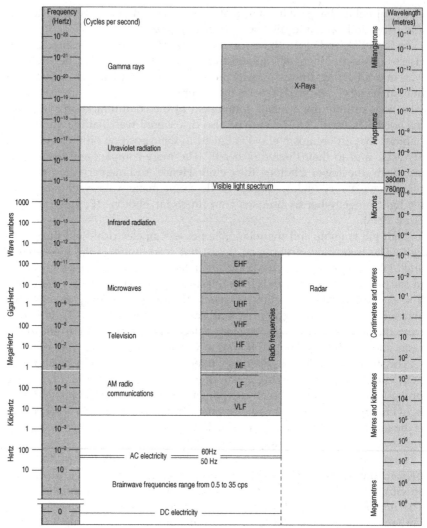

Fig 4.1 The electromagnetic spectrum. With permission from Sylver N 2008 The Holistic Handbook of Sauna Therapy. Townsend Letter, February/March 2008.

(called 'interference'), the way in which they overlap influences the impact of the union. If the wave patterns are in sync – that is, they are in phase with each other, the impact is additive and will be reflected in the new waveform having an amplitude that is greater than each individual wave's amplitude – like increases like. Two waves are said to be in phase when they are both, in effect, peaking or troughing at the same time, even if they have different frequencies or amplitudes. Getting 'in phase' is getting in sync (McTaggart 2002). This type of encounter is called 'constructive interference' (Fig. 4.3). If the wave patterns are opposite – that is, one is peaking while the other is troughing, the two wave patterns will tend to cancel each other out – opposites balance. This type of union is called 'destructive interference'.

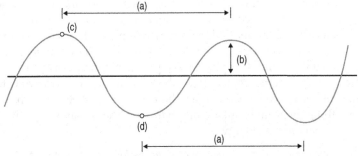

Fig 4.2 Wave patterns. (a) Wavelength; (b) amplitude; (c) peak; (d) trough.

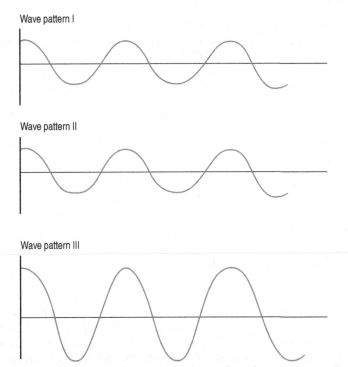

Wave pattern I

Wave pattern II

Wave pattern III

Fig 4.3 Constructive interference. Wave III is the additive effect of wave I plus wave II.

CELLULAR COMMUNICATION

Cellular communication is initiated by endogenous and exogenous factors; between individuals and their environment, between individuals, within all aspects of an individual, and between organs, tissues, and cells. Some signals are tangible, some intangible; all have an energetic wave pattern with their own rhythm and frequency.

The communication functions of the nervous, endocrine, and cardiovascular systems were the basis for understanding cellular communication, yet there was always the sense that there was something more. For example, there are no nerves connecting muscles with the arterioles that supply them with oxygen and nutrients. A piece of the puzzle was uncovered in the 1980s when it was discovered that part of this communication was due to the exchange of nitric oxide. Even then there was the recognition that there was something even more intangible than gas. The missing piece is vibrational wave patterns of energy.

Energy fields are available to nature as a means for providing even faster control than a diffusible gas with a 10-second lifetime. Some energy fields travel at the speed of light; others are instantaneous. For nature to have left these communication modalities out of its 'bag of tricks' is highly unlikely (Oschman 2003).

What determines cellular communication and life is constant vibration and interaction of all components. Life is vibrational energy, movement is life; if no movement there is death (Emoto 2004).

The intangible signals such as sound, light, thoughts, touch, magnetic energy, and electronic conduction, affect cellular communication. For example,

We now know that light is a major component of the vibratory communication system of the body, because such vibrations have been both predicted on the basis of fundamental biophysical theory and measured by sensitive devices (Popp et al 1992, Oschman & Oschman 1997).

Each color vibrates in specific wave patterns and at a specific frequency. 'In the visible spectrum, red, with the longest frequency, has the lowest vibration rate, and violet, with the shortest frequency, has the highest vibration rate' (Steinberg 2007). Colors have a tremendous impact on health; including, vision, mood, energy level, appetite, sleeping, and even the functioning of organs and tissues (Elvin 2007, Steinberg 2007).

Sound impacts individuals in all forms; such as spoken words, an individual's own thoughts, words you hear from others, the sounds of nature, the environment, and music (Sylver 2008). An individual's voice itself has a range of speaking, a specific tone, frequency, rate and pace of speech. Individuals convey energy by speaking, not just in the words that they choose, but in how they say it. Sound patterns impact health, whether we can hear them or not, and each sound is heard differently depending on the instrument that is being used. For example, all music notes are found to vibrate at specific frequency and have a specified wave length. You can hear the same vibration, although displayed differently, based on the instrument that is playing a specific note.

When we expand our understanding of signaling to the tangible and intangible, we recognize that initiation of cellular communication occurs in response to all stimuli and it can no longer be thought of as a linear causality process based on physical molecules. As more sensitive pieces of equipment are designed to explore the intangible forms of energetic vibration, we will have a deeper understanding of how it affects cellular communication, and how it can be used in the treatment of diseases.

Cellular communication is considered healthy when there is harmony and coherence. Harmony refers to the attunement and consistency of energetic vibration throughout the body. Perfect coherence is an optimum state just between chaos and order. To maintain health you need to take in the correct quantity and quality of energy (light) from various sources such as food, sunlight, thoughts, emotions, bodywork, etc., and be able to filter it, respond to it, and use it appropriately. You also need to have all systems in the body working coherently, in harmony, alignment and in sync. The coherence between the different aspects of the body influences the movement and communication of the whole system. In other words, ill health occurs when systemic communication breaks down and when a person's waves are out of sync with each other and with their surroundings.

THE ROLE OF WATER

All cellular communication uses water and water is the primary vehicle for the transmission of chemicals, hormones, and nutrients throughout the body. Water is the medium responsible for sending and amplifying energetic wave patterns (McTaggart 2002, Oschman 2003).

Water is the natural medium for all cells. A fetus is about 99% water. When we are born we are about 90% and as adults we are about 70% water. In every cell there is one molecule of protein for every ten thousand molecules of water and it is water that holds the double helix together. The full understanding of the importance of water often is overlooked. Water is extremely adaptable; it can convert easily between a solid, a liquid, and a gas.

The ability of water to copy, memorize, and carry energetic signals and messages was shown in the 1980s by the researcher Jacques Benveniste. In an experiment, he exposed ordinary water to the recorded signals of acetylcholine and ovalbumin and then transmitted the recordings via a computer to another lab. The recordings were then introduced to isolated guinea pig hearts. The effects of the digitized water were identical to effects produced on the heart by the actual substances themselves (Benveniste et al 1997). This experiment and others like it, although controversial, provide insight into the importance of water in cellular communication and the ability of water to duplicate and transmit the energy frequencies of a substance. The ability of water to copy and memorize information is also the theory behind the plussing, or potentiation process that is used in homeopathy (Vithoulkas 1980).

The work of Masaru Emoto, in *The Hidden Messages in Water* (2001), further emphasized the unlimited ability of the water to copy and store information. He demonstrated that thoughts and words have the ability to change the crystallized formation of water. Emoto wrapped a piece of paper with words typed on it around a bottle of water. He then froze the water, and then cut the frozen cubes of water and took pictures of the ice crystals. What he discovered was that when the words or thoughts are positive the crystal formations are complete, symmetrical and colorful; when they are negative the formations are incomplete, asymmetrical and dull (Emoto 2001). There are some scientists who question the validity of Emoto's work, but if, or when, it is accepted to be true the possibilities and significance are immense, especially when you consider that human beings are primarily water.

Human beings as complex, dynamic systems of energy

Thoughts and words, whether spoken or written, initiate a wave pattern and influence their environment. Water has a tremendous capability to store memories and different wave patterns, vibrations, and frequencies. Water is the conductor and the amplifier for life. It is the transmission medium for the body and it is meant to continuously move. 'Water in a river remains pure because it is moving. When water becomes trapped, it dies. Therefore, water must constantly be circulated. The water – or blood – in the bodies of the sick is usually stagnant. When blood stops flowing, the body starts to decay (Emoto 2001). Water might be the most overlooked aspect of preventative health care and might be the most valuable treatment tool that we can use.

MOVEMENT

If there is no movement, there is no life. The difference between health and disease lies in the relative freedom, flexibility and coherence of the energetic wave pulsations throughout the body. All pulsations of life energy occur in patterns of expansion and contraction, centrifugal and centripetal, or involution and evolution.

The movement of various components of the body follows a closed loop effect, yet this movement is not autonomous – it is affected by every other system and wave vibration of the body. These closed loop movements have a source, where energy flows out from and then returns. All physiological responses in the body follow this pattern. For example, the heart pumps and sends blood to the body and that blood returns to the heart, there is a continual inhalation and exhalation of breath, the cerebrospinal fluid flows from the ventricles of the brain to the coccyx and then back, and contraction and relaxation of muscles. When this natural rhythm and flow of movement is blocked it results in a disruption to the health of the organism.

The elemental properties of air, fire, and water, as well Yin and Yang, are characterized by their type of movement. Air moves in a more east–west direction, water in a north–south direction, fire has a spiral wave pattern, Yin moves inward or in a centripetal fashion, whereas Yang moves outward or centrifugally (Fig. 4.4). These different movement patterns create a continual flow of energy throughout the body (Burger 1998, Pole 2006).

COMPLEX SYSTEMS

The new scientific understanding of life is that all living systems – organisms, social systems, ecosystems – are complex systems. All systems are interconnected and interdependent; no system can be understood in isolation. Complex systems theory recognizes that the properties of the whole are the essential properties, not the properties of the parts.

Systems thinking is 'contextual' which is the opposite of analytical thinking. Analysis means taking something apart in order to understand it; systems thinking means putting it into the context of a larger whole (Capra 1988).

Every part of a system is able to influence every other part and this understanding is destroyed when a system is dissected into isolated elements. This

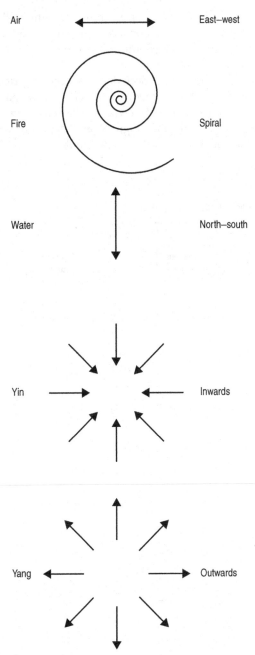

Air   East–west

Fire   Spiral

Water   North–south

Yin   Inwards

Yang   Outwards

Fig 4.4 Directions of movement.

intrinsic nature of systems is able to create outcomes that defy our current physiological understandings. For example, thinking about a pattern of movements sets up a corresponding pattern of electrical activity in the nervous system, even though no actual movements are taking place; when sport activities are rehearsed mentally it improves performance; when dancers or musicians perform sometimes the electrical signals cease, even though the performer is still moving (Oschman 2003). Every part of an individual is linked and all parts move as one. For example, thoughts influence physical structure, emotions stimulate functional changes in the body, and structural changes impact the internal functioning of organs (Fig. 4.5). Every part is dependent and influenced by every other.

The concept of systemic interconnectedness is a central principle of naturopathic medicine and of all eastern medicines, such as Ayurvedic, Chinese, and Unani medicine. The concept is not new, but what has changed over time is the research to support it and the language and depth of understanding of how all parts relate and work together as one unit.

(a) "Old" Conventional Model of Human Beings

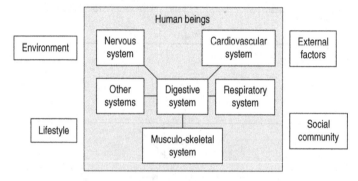

(b) "New" Complex Systems Model of Human Beings

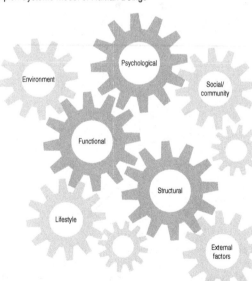

Fig 4.5 Complex systems. (a) 'Old' conventional model of human beings. Human beings were thought of from a reductionist point of view. Each part was viewed and treated separately, and human beings were felt to be separate from their external environment. (b) 'New' complex systems model of human beings. Human beings are complex systems. Each part interacts and is influenced by every other part, including the external environment and other people. The parts are linked, like a 'cogwheel'. Changes in one part create movement in every other part.

Self-organizing

Human beings are self-organizing systems that maintain a complex pattern of organization; a configuration of relationships within a living matrix. Self-organizing systems have hierarchical patterns (Fig. 4.6) that are multi-leveled, interrelated, and interdependent. Each system functions as a whole (suprasystem), yet consists of smaller and smaller parts (subsystems), each part with its own function and structure. These smaller parts are subsystems of the greater system, the suprasystem (Capra 1996). It is the relationship between the parts that is relevant and that determines the state of health of the whole system.

If you look at human beings as the suprasystem, then the subsystems include each of the organ systems: immune, cardiovascular, endocrine, nervous, musculoskeletal, etc. Every organ system can be broken down into smaller and smaller subsystems that function as a network. For example the cardiovascular system contains the heart, veins, arteries, and blood. Every subsystem is equally important, is integral to the health of an individual, and is interrelated with every other system.

Human beings are a subsystem of other systems. For example, human beings are a subsystem of the greater universal system, just as animals, trees, water, and air are also subsystems of this system. Human beings are a subsystem of a social system which includes community, family, work, friends, etc. Every aspect of life is a part of many different systems, all of which are interrelated and connected.

The concept of self-organizing is a basis of traditional medical systems and naturopathic medicine. For example, according to Chinese medicine,

> The self-organizing process is a product of the interaction of qi (the dynamic impulse, architect of form and function), jing (the fundamental substance, origin of our nature), and ming (the urge toward actualization and fulfillment, destiny) (Beinfield & Korngold 1991).

This self-organizing capability occurs in response to adversity, and in the process of growing, thriving, and living.

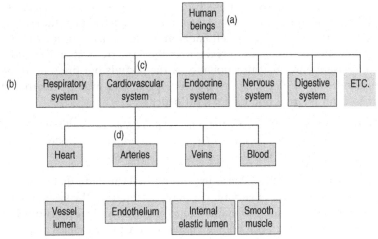

Fig 4.6 Hierarchical look at human beings. (a) Human beings as the suprasystem; (b) clinical systems as the suprasystem and a subsystem of human beings; (c) cardiovascular system as the suprasystem and a subsystem of clinical systems; (d) arteriole system as the suprasystem and a subsystem of the cardiovascular system.

Open systems

In order for human beings to survive they have to maintain a continuous exchange of energy and matter with their environment. For example, there is a continuous need for nutrients such as air, water, and food, and the body, while processing the nutrients, continually produces and eliminates waste products back into the environment.

> *In fact, everything which exists in the external universe has its counterpart in a living being's own personal internal universe...The flow of nutrients into and wastes out of body cells also characterizes the continuous flow of nutrients and wastes into and out of plants, animals and humans (Svoboda 1988).*

The health of each system is dependent on the health of every system. Human beings consume food and water and breathe the air that is in their environment. The amount of life energy and the health of each part affect the health of each human being. Human beings are in constant interplay with their surroundings. Life is not about the isolated survival of each individual, but about the interplay and interaction of everyone with everything. Maybe the apprehension for recognizing and adopting this new understanding of life comes from the realization that to do so increases the understanding that we must take responsibility for ourselves and for the world.

Self-renewal

Self-organizing systems are able to continuously renew and recycle their components while maintaining the integrity of the overall structures (Capra 1988). Human beings adapt and compensate to internal and external stimuli as they continuously grow, develop, and repair each part of their system. When an individual has the essential components to life, such as, food, nutrients, movement, water, sleep, rest, fresh air, loving relationships, etc the body has the inherent ability to self-renew and maintain a dynamic state of health.

This dynamic state was originally called homeostasis, and is currently referred to as the homeodynamic state. Homeodynamics takes into consideration the energetic concepts of cellular communication, quantum theory and irreversible thermodynamics. It recognizes that communication is based on a mutual causality and that functionality of the body is not program driven.

Human beings are open systems that respond and provide internal feedback based on internal and external influences.

> *Unlike closed systems, which settle into a state of thermal equilibrium, open systems maintain themselves far from equilibrium in this 'steady state' characterized by continual flow and change (Capra 1988).*

The presence of feedback loops implies mutual causality that is the recognition that there are many variables at play. Each part of the system requires certain nutrients or stimuli to maintain its functions, and all functions fluctuate between an upper and a lower limit. When the variables required to maintain functioning of one part of the system are imbalanced or disrupted, this results in changes in other parts of the system.

The variables that can disrupt the homeodynamic state of any part of the system include nutritional deficiencies, the accumulation of toxins, emotional stress, poor posture, a lack of sleep or any other excesses or deficiencies in lifestyle and environmental factors.

At a certain point in time the adaptive homeostatic mechanisms break down, and frank illness – disease – appears. At this time the situation has modified from homeostasis to heterostasis, and at this time the body needs help – treatment (Chaitow et al 2002).

When there is a disruption to the homeodynamic state, the body adapts or compensates by the stimulation of inherent corrective mechanisms. When the body is unable to re-establish a homeodynamic balance, signs and symptoms will manifest on some level. The aim of naturopathic treatment is to improve the overall functioning of the body as a whole, as there is recognition that the site of discomfort is not always the area that caused the disruption.

Mutual causality

Mutual causality recognizes that there might be a relationship between two things, yet the outcome is contextual and variable, based on multidirectional influences, feedback from other parts, and rule-governed processes that control the system. This variability leads to increased adaptability as the more variables that there are in a system, the more mechanisms that can potentially provide redundancy. Mutual causality provides for an integrated understanding of life and is better able to explain how the body handles and assimilates the many different influences that it encounters than can linear causality (see Fig. 4.7). 'Reality appears as a dynamically interdependent process. All factors, mental and physical, subsist in a web of mutual causal interaction, with no element or essence held to be immutable or autonomous' (Macy 1991).

Mutual causality explains the uniqueness of individuals. The impact of accidents or stressful situations is not the same for every person, individuals with the same disease often have different symptoms, diseases progress differently

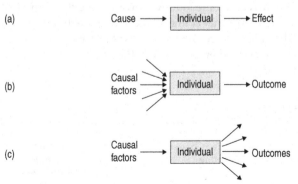

Fig 4.7 Causality (a) Linear causality: there is a direct correlation between cause and effect; (b) mutual causality: a single outcome can be due to the interaction of various factors; (c) mutual causality: a single factor can result in various outcomes.

Human beings as complex, dynamic systems of energy

for each person, the impact of the same symptom is experienced differently, etc. The same food for one person can be medicine; for another poison. The same treatment can have opposite effects on different individuals. Life is complex, human beings are complex. Mutual causality recognizes this complexity, the interrelationship of individuals to their environment, and the uniqueness of individuals.

Self-transcendence

Complex self-organizing systems are able to self-renew and have the ability for self-transcendence – 'the ability to reach out creatively beyond physical and mental boundaries in the processes of learning, development, and evolution' (Capra 1988). Self-transcendence involves individuals conceiving themselves as an integral part of the universe as a whole. It is about moving beyond the physical and the ego, and knowing the inner spirit essence of life, it is about seeing the world from a universal perspective. At the heart of self-transcendence is a spiritual concept that looks at the true meaning of life and the infinite consciousness.

In most religions and in many traditional and alternative medical theories there is an understanding, a belief, that there is a spirit essence, greater than any individual. Recognizing that each person is an integral part of a larger whole is beneficial to health.

People were more likely to succeed if, instead of believing in a distinction between themselves and the world, and seeing individual people and things as isolated and divisible, they viewed everything as a connected continuum of interactions – and also if they understood that there were other ways to communicate than through the usual channels (Braud 1975).

The concept of a collective consciousness is about believing in an energetic force that is greater than any individual. 'Consciousness was a global phenomenon that occurred everywhere in the body and not simply in our brains. Consciousness, at its most basic, was coherent light' (McTaggart 2002). The collective consciousness is the force that connects everyone together, it explains the knowingness that is between close friends and family members, the ability of the mind to create dreams of future events, and the instinct that drives people to move towards one thing and to avoid something else. It is the force that connects individuals with the subtangible physical world. The collective consciousness explains the ability of the people to influence objects and other people whether they are in close contact or a wide distance apart.

REFERENCES

Beinfield H, Korngold E 1991 Between Heaven and Earth, a Guide to Chinese Medicine. Ballantine Wellspring, New York

Benveniste J, Jurgens P, Hsueh W, Aissa J 1997 Transaltantic transfer of dignitized antigen signal by telephone link. J Allergy Clin Immunol 99:175 In McTaggart L 2002 The Field. HarperCollins, London

Braud WG 1975 Psi-conducive states. J Communication 25(1):142–152. In McTaggart L 2002 The Field. HarperCollins, London

Burger B 1998 Esoteric Anatomy, the Body as Consciousness. North Atlantic Books, California

Burr H 1972 The Fields of Life. Ballantine, New York

Capra F 1996 The Web of Life. Anchor Books, New York

Capra F 1988 The Turning Point, Science, Society and the Rising Culture. Bantaum Books, Toronto

Chaitow L, Bradley D, Gilbert C 2002 Multidisciplinary Approaches to Breathing Pattern Disorders. Churchill Livingstone, Edinburgh

Elvin C 2007 Complementary therapies: using color in care. Nursing & Residential Care 9(9):417–419

Emoto M 2001 The Hidden Messages in Water. Beyond Words, New York

Emoto M 2004 Love Thyself, the Message from Water III. Hay House, Carlsbad

Haisch B, Rueda A, Puthoff HE 1994 Beyond E=mc2: A First Glimpse of a Universe Without Mass. The Sciences

Hunt VV 1996 Infinite Mind, Science of Human Vibrations of Consciousness. Malibu Publishing, California

Macy J 1991 Mutual Causality in Buddhism and General Systems Theory. State University Press, New York

McTaggart L 2002 The Field, The Quest for the Secret Force of the Universe. HarperCollins, London

Oschman JL 2003 Energy Medicine in Therapeutics and Human Performance. Butterworth-Heinemann, Edinburgh

Oschman JL, Oschman NH 1997 Book review and commentary: biological coherence and response to external stimuli, edited by H Fröhlich, Springer-Verlag, Berlin. In Oschman JL 2003 Energy Medicine in Therapeutics and Human Performance. Butterworth-Heinemann, Edinburgh

Pole S 2006 Ayurvedic Medicine, the Principles of Traditional Practice. Churchill Livingstone, Philadelphia

Popp FA, Li KH, Gu Q 1992 Recent Advances in Biophoton Research and its Applications. World Scientific, Singapore

Steinberg H 2007 A new 'light' on color light therapy: visual color therapy and the effect on disease conditions. Townsend Letter

Svoboda R 1988 Prakruti, your Ayurvedic Constitution. Geocom, New Mexico

Sylver N 2008 Healing with Electromedicine and Sound Therapies, part one. Townsend Letter February/March 93–99

Vithoulkas G 1980 The Science of Homeopathy. Grove Press, New York

FURTHER READING

Arntz W, Chase B, Vicente M 2005 What the Bleep do we Know. Health Communications, Florida

Cannon WB 1932 The Wisdom of the Body. WW Norton, New York

Castaneda C 1998 The Active Side of Infinity. Harper Perennial, New York

Cohen S, Popp FA 1997 Biophoton emission of the human body. J Photochem Photobiol Biology 40:187–189

Legge D 1997 Close to the Bone, The Treatment of Musculo-Skeletal Disorder With Acupuncture and Other Traditional Chinese Medicine, second edition. Sydney College Press, Australia

Louise C 2008 Systems Theory and Naturopathic Philosophy The Healing Power of Nature: The Foundations of Naturopathic Medicine. Elsevier, Missouri

Magner L 1992 A history of medicine. Dekker, New York

McGuiness L 2007 The Healing Power of Color. Positive Health November 14–16

Moor FB, FB, Peterson SC, Manwell EM, Nobel MC, Muench G 1964 Manual of Hydrotherapy and Massage. Pacific Press, Ontario

Rucker R 2005 Infinity and the Mind, the Science and Philosophy of the Infinite. Princeton University Press, Princeton

Sills F 1989 The Polarity Process, Energy as a Healing Art. Element, Dorset

Smith FF 1986 Inner Bridges, a Guide to Energy Movement and Body Structures. Humanics New Age, Georgia

Stone RB 1989 The Secret Life of Your Cells. Whitford Press, Philadelphia

Talbot M 1991 The Holographic Universe. Harper Perennial, New York

Turner RN 2000 Naturopathic Medicine, Treating the Whole Person. Thorsons, UK

Wolinsky S 1994 The Tao of Chaos. Bramble Books, Connecticut

Human beings as complex, dynamic systems of energy

CHAPTER 5
Symptom patterns

A truly holistic and integrated medical approach is achieved by using a common framework and language for the assessment, diagnosis, and treatment of health and disease, and by using this same framework to describe everything in nature. Traditional medical systems use consistent terms to describe the qualities and characteristics of seasons, nature, food, herbs, times of day, stages of life, body composition and temperaments, and to describe symptoms and diseases. This consistency in terminology aids greatly in understanding and assessing the relationship between human beings and their environment and lifestyle.

All symptoms display a pattern that can be classified according to specific qualities and attributes. Assessing symptoms takes practice and patience. For many, it is a new window and way of looking at health and disease; it involves observing all parts of life based on their qualities and attributes and understanding how everything interacts and influences each other. Exploring symptoms does not exclude the knowledge and learning that is gained from the conventional assessment model; it adds to the breadth and depth of the understanding and it provides a link between the symptoms and their cause. In naturopathic medicine there is the recognition each individual is unique and there is meaning and purpose for why symptoms and diseases appear. The exploration of symptom patterns brings reason and order back into health and disease, it appreciates and recognizes the complexity and intricacy of the human body, and the interrelationships among people, their environment, and external factors.

The body displays symptoms of disharmony and exhaustion in many different ways. This book explores the patterns of internal and external, excess and deficiency, Yin–Yang, the five elements, and symbolism of body parts. The examples below provide generalizations of how the qualities and attributes of patterns manifest. Understanding patterns is an intrinsic art and science with many contributing factors and variables. It is important to realize that the examples are provided as a guide, not as an absolute. When assessing the patterns, the aim is to observe how the nature of the symptoms and the locations of the symptoms reveal a story that relates the patient in front of you. As a practitioner, be cautious about leading or labeling the patterns. For example, frustrated, irritable, angry, are labels. During the assessment you are looking for the qualities and characteristics that convey the meaning.

EXTERNAL/INTERNAL

The pattern of internal versus external refers to whether the focus of a patient is on the self or others. Like all aspects of energy, the concept of internal and external is a continuum. It is the balance between internal and external that results in health. The concept of internal/external is a component of the Yin–Yang theory. It is listed separately as a way of highlighting its significance in the therapeutic assessment process. It is also the first pattern that usually becomes apparent during the initial therapeutic encounter: you hear a patient's focus in their language, in their stories and how they reveal their thoughts, motivation and choices.

Externally focused patients are preoccupied with outside factors – what they do for a living, how many children they have, their job, and their responsibility to others. Those that are externally focused become concerned with their health when it affects their inability to fulfill their responsibilities to others. Predominantly, externally focused patients have less awareness of their psychological, functional, or structural state; for example, the frequency of bowel movements, the cause of bruises, the presence of muscle tension, even their own thoughts, or what they recently ate. They are less aware of the timing, intensity, and duration of physical symptoms or how these symptoms relate to their lifestyle.

Decisions are based on external commitments; for example, they will hold off on taking that needed vacation because there is a big project at work, or they find that they have no time to work-out because they are busy taking care of everyone else. Externally focused patients put others first and themselves last. They have a tendency to be easily affected by what is going on with family, friends, their job, their responsibilities, their community, and the environment.

A patient who is *internally focused* is preoccupied with self – how they are feeling, what part of their body is bothering them, their aches and pains, their hardships, and how they are affected by others. There is increased personal responsibility for the situations and outcomes in their life. There is also more awareness of the psychological, functional, and/or structural aspects of their health, often resulting in a heightened attention to and concern for any signs or symptoms. An internal focus, to a degree, is needed when a patient is looking at shifting to a higher state of health, as it is valuable to bring your energy 'home' in order to heal.

Internally focused patients see the world from the perspective of self. When situations or events happen, the impact is personal, it is about them, their ability to fulfill their dreams and passions, and how the situations or events have affected their health. For example, if a patient with an internal focus loses their job they are more likely to see it as a reflection of something that they did wrong, or as a personal opportunity to change and grow; as opposed to thinking that it is about something external, such as an unfair manager or a down-turn in the market.

Internal and external intentions look at a person's psychological state and recognize that these states are mirrored in the physical body (Fig. 5.1). The closer the symptom is to the midline or medial aspect of the body part the more it is about 'self'. The more symptoms are lateral, or on the periphery the more they are about a patient's reaction to something external or someone else. For example, Fig. 5.2 indicates an external stance and Fig. 5.3 an internal sitting posture.

Symptoms that manifest on the face tend to be associated with external factors or when a patient is concerned with how they are perceived by others, as the face is the aspect of the body that is the most visible to the outside world. With symptoms there often is a blending of both. The extremities, for example, tend to represent our relationship to the external world. The arms are used to give and receive; with the legs we move forward through life. Even within the extremities there is a medial and lateral component. The inner aspect of the thigh and the inside of the arm are more medial

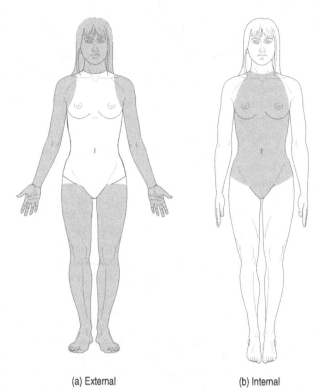

(a) External   (b) Internal

Fig 5.1 Internal/external. (a) External. The focus of a person's energy and attention is on external events and situations. Symptoms most commonly appear on the periphery and lateral aspects of the body. (b) Internal. The focus of a person's attention is on the self and how situations impact them personally. Symptoms most commonly appear in medial and central aspects of the body.

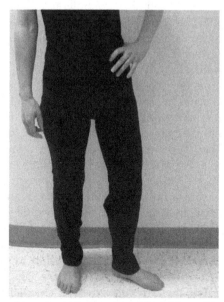

Fig 5.2 External stance. Note the external rotation of the left leg and foot.

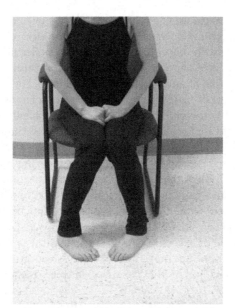

Fig 5.3 Internal posture. Notice the internal rotation of the legs and feet and the arms.

and tend to be affected when the concern is more about how an external factor, person or event affects us personally.

Case 5.1

A 45-year-old female has the chief complaint of Raynaud's syndrome. Her hands and feet become very cold in cold weather and when she is nervous. She reports having low self-esteem and being fearful of making mistakes and looking stupid in front of other people. When she is upset she keeps it to herself. She has a moderate build, and presents with rounded shoulders, forward head posture, and a slight internal rotation of her arms and feet when standing. Overall her frame is collapsed and her energy is internally focused. The treatment involved acupuncture to 'call the energy' to the periphery, warming foods and herbs, and counseling to address the low self-esteem. The acupuncture, food, and herbs lessened the intensity of the coldness. As the patient's self-esteem increased and as she learned to share more of her thoughts and feeling with others the Raynaud symptoms were resolved.

EXCESS AND DEFICIENCY

The body is always processing and interacting with its internal and external environment as it continuously regulates, compensates, and distributes the ongoing influx of stimuli, sensations, nutrients, thoughts, etc. Health is maintained when the influx of stimuli and nutrients meets the needs of the body. When there is an imbalance between what is needed and what is received, symptoms manifest. Any manifestation of a symptom can be quantitatively looked at on the continuum of excess to deficiency; even other energetic concepts, such as internal/external, Yin–Yang, and the elements are often expressed quantitatively based on excesses and deficiencies. What exactly is too much or too little depends on the unique constitution and susceptibilities of each individual at any specific point and time. For example, a healthy individual with a lot of 'fire' will often desire and tolerate spicy food, more than an individual with very little fire. On the other hand, the healthy 'fiery' individual may find that when they are overwhelmed they do best to avoid spicy food.

It is common for a person to have factors in their life that contribute to a state of excess and others that contribute to a state of deficiency. For example, excess coffee and food, long hours at work, too much time in front of a computer; coupled with a deficiency in sleep, movement, and exercise, and too little fresh air. Sometimes, the reason why a specific behaviour or a food causes a state of excess is because of when it was done or consumed. For example, an individual may find that they sleep great when they exercise during the day, but if they exercise later in the evening they have difficulty falling asleep.

The overall impact on health is based on the accumulation of all factors and their context. Like increases like, and opposites decrease each other. For example, hot spicy food, warm sunny weather, bright colored clothing, the emotions irritability and frustration all increase fire. Each of these alone might not be excessive but the effects are additive and together they cause the body to be in a state of excess. Individual factors will display a state of excess or deficiency as will the overall state of a person's health. Also, whenever there is a state of excess in one aspect of an individual, another aspect often becomes deficient as a way of compensating or maintaining internal balance. For example, the consumption of excess coffee results in an inability to sleep, or when excess worry results in constipation (decreased movement in the bowels) (Frawley 1989, Maciocia 1989).

The misuse, under or over use, and abuse of the senses also contributes to excesses and deficiencies. The senses are the main avenue for taking in information and experiencing life. Constant visual and auditory stimulation overwhelms the body. For example, many people relax after a long day's work by sitting in front of the television; the eyes and ears are still being stimulated. With the tremendous increase of electronic communication, the ability and opportunity to speak has decreased. Many people eat in such a hurry that they seldom taste their food, hence negatively impacting the body's ability to produce the digestive and pancreatic exocrine secretions that are needed.

Excess

Excess is about too much. It can occur because of excesses in specific dietary and lifestyle behaviors, such as too much food, alcohol, cigarettes, anger, sadness, exercise, television, work, etc. A state of excess is caused by an imbalance between what you take in (digest or absorb) and what you let go of (secrete or express); both literally and figuratively. For the body to maintain health there needs to be a balance between the two. Excess also can occur by taking in too much from the external environment – excessive noise, light, stress, responsibilities, possessions, etc.

When in a state of excess, the circulation of energy is impacted and becomes congested or blocked. Excess manifests in symptoms such as intense, forceful movements, loud and full voice, intensity in thoughts or emotions, heavy breathing, pains that are worse with pressure, swelling and inflammation, or an increase in weight or size. A thick coat on the tongue and a rapid strong pulse indicate a state of excess (Kaptchuk 1983, Maciocia 1989). There also can be an excess of hormones, enzymes, stomach acid, and fluid. On a structural level, excess manifests as stiffness or heaviness. In order to treat an excess state, it is necessary to decrease the factor(s) contributing to the excess, and to promote the normal movement of energy or bodily fluids to the areas concerned.

Deficiency

There are two main causes of deficiency: an insufficiency of nutrients or energy needed for optimal functioning, and a state of deficiency brought on due to a state of exhaustion after being in a state of excess for too long. An example of the former is a patient with a poor diet, not enough sleep or relaxation, lack of exercise, lack of water, lack of nurturing, and not feeling safe or loved. An example of the latter is a patient where the excesses in lifestyle have exhausted the body's reserves attempting to compensate and adapt and the body starts to break down. Most chronic conditions are due to a combination of both.

In a deficiency state, an individual's healing potential is compromised, and their resistance is low. The general symptoms of deficiency include white or pale complexion, fatigue, weakness and loss of strength, poor spirits, shallow breathing, pain relieved by pressure, too tired to talk, a low and feeble voice, excessive or spontaneous perspiration, and incontinence and insufficient hormones, enzymes, stomach acid or fluids such as urine, feces, or sweat. Deficiency causes a breakdown in tissues, organs, muscles, and structure. The tongue is pale and thin and the pulse feels weak (Maciocia 1998).

YIN–YANG

Yin–Yang is the single most important and distinctive concept of Chinese medicine (Table 5.1). This concept is extremely simple, yet very profound. It can be used to explain the quantitative and qualitative aspects of nature, physiology, pathology, and treatments. It is based on the flow of energy between two extremes. Yin–Yang is a continuum without borders or boundaries; it represents opposite yet complementary qualities.

Every phenomenon in the universe alternates through a cyclical movement of peaks and bases, and the alteration of Yin and Yang is the motive force of its change and development. Day changes into night, summer into winter, growth into decay and vice versa (Maciocia 1989).

Table 5.1   Yin–Yang (Kaptchuk 1983, Maciocia 1989, Beinfield & Korngold 1991)

Yang energy	Yin energy
Superior, top-down	Inferior, bottom-up
Exterior, inside-out, centrifugal	Interior, outside-in, centripetal
Back	Front
Posterior-lateral surface	Anterior-medial surface
Front of the body – right side	Front of the body – left side
Back of the body – left side	Back of the body – right side
Left side of face	Right side of face
Superficial aspects of the body	Deeper aspects and organs in the body
Above the waist	Below the waist
Organs: gallbladder, stomach, small intestines, large intestines, urinary bladder and triple burner	Organs: heart, lungs, spleen, liver and kidneys
Breath – exhalation	Breath – inhalation
Qi, defensive Qi	Blood-body fluids, nutritive Qi
Masculine qualities	Feminine qualities
Purpose: function, activity, to receive, break down and absorb, generate, and to transform, transport and change	Purpose: structure, rest, to give, grow, regulate, conserve and store energy, spirit, fluids and blood
Characteristics: motion, outgoing, transforming, responsible, expressive, steady, aggressive, action-oriented, large firm and fleshy body, coarse features, high energy	Characteristics: yielding, nourishing, passive, feeling, maintenance, intuitive, receptive, creative, listening, gentle, flaccid body, delicate features
Signs and symptoms: excess, hot, dry, hard, rapid, expansion, heavy, restlessness, loud, stiffness, forceful movements, likes to stretch out, respiration is full and deep, sense of fullness, strong odor, pressure aggravates discomfort, hypertensive	Signs and symptoms: deficiency, cold, wet, soft, slow, quiet, contraction, sleepiness, weak, lack of strength, tired, likes to be curled up, excretions are thin, shortness of breath, sense of emptiness, pressure relieves discomfort, hypotensive
Push, extensor muscles	Pull, flexor muscles
Pathway into the material world	Pathway toward spirit.
Light, brightness	Darkness, shade
Sun, the cosmos	Moon, Earth
Summer, spring	Winter, autumn
East, south	West, north
To balance begin at the core and work outwards	To balance use heat, begin at the extremities and move to the core
Often associated with acute illnesses, rapid onset	Often associated with chronic illnesses, gradual onset

The manifestation of Yin–Yang

Every component of an individual contains both aspects of Yin and Yang. These are seldom present in a 50/50 proportion, yet instead in a dynamic and constantly changing balance that is unique for each person (Kaptchuk 1983). For example, an individual who is more outgoing, aggressive, and strong would be considered Yang; whereas someone who was more nurturing, quiet, and of smaller build would be considered Yin. From a physiological point of view, this constant balancing is seen in the body's innate ability to regulate sweating, urination, temperature of the body, breathing, etc.

(Maciocia 1989). If Yin or Yang qualities are extended beyond their normal range of functioning, pathological changes will occur.

Diseases that have the qualities of heat, restlessness, and fullness indicate a preponderance of Yang; whereas, diseases that are characterized by weakness and coldness indicate more of a Yin condition. Acute diseases are often due to an excess of Yang. Chronic diseases, for the most part, are due to a Yin deficiency state (Maciocia 1989, Beinfield & Korngold 1991). The presence of a more predominant Yin or Yang is also apparent when the symptoms have a sidedness, a tendency to be more right or left, or more front versus the back. For example, a patient with pain and weakness in their left shoulder, a sensitive left hip, weak knees worse on the left, and an ear infection that started on the left side, would have a Yin imbalance. This imbalance might be caused by a lack of Yin qualities in a person's life – e.g., nurturing, rest, creativity – or it can be due to an excess of Yang qualities – e.g., excessive work, exercise, alcohol; which in turn weaken Yin.

The presence of Yin–Yang can be thought of as a balance board (Fig. 5.4) that is in constant movement; as one increases the other decreases. When Yang is too high, Yin is deficient; when Yin is too high, Yang is deficient. Imbalances can also occur as a result of deficiency of either Yin or Yang. In this case, the predominant quality will lead to an apparent excess of other. For example, a deficiency of Yang will result in an apparent excess of Yin; a deficiency of Yin will result in an apparent excess of Yang.

Symptom patterns

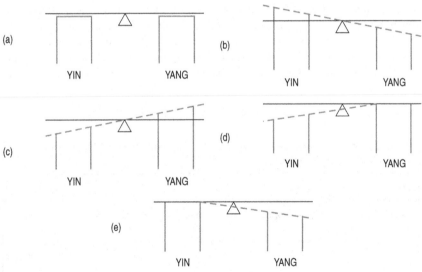

Fig 5.4 Yin–Yang balance. (a) Balance of Yin and Yang; (b) Yin excess; (c) Yang excess; (d) Yin deficiency; (e) Yang deficiency.

FIVE ELEMENTS

Ayurvedic, Chinese, and Unani medicine as well as polarity therapy have elements, and their qualities, as the foundation for how they explain life, health and disease. For the purposes of this book, the elemental qualities of ether, air, fire, water, and earth which are taken from Ayurvedic and Unani medicine and polarity therapy will be explored. These qualities represent the quantitative aspects of all matter, both organic and inorganic (Lad 1998). As described in Chapter 2, Ayurvedic and Unani medicine uses the qualities of the elements to represent specific doshas and humors, respectively. The purpose of this book is to explore the concepts of each element individually, recognizing that there are always at least two elements or qualities interacting to create a pattern.

Everything in nature and life is composed of these five elements, in varying proportions; just as there are shades of color, each one blending into the other. Each element has specific qualities and attributes that create its unique vibration. This vibration manifests in many forms: color, sound, emotion, thoughts, structure etc. For example, the fire element is yellow in color, it is heard in loud staccato music, it is felt in the heat of the summer; fire food is hot and spicy; irritability and frustration are examples of fire emotions, as are passion, motivation, and enthusiasm; and a fire build is muscular (Burger 1998, Lloyd 2006). The quality of earth in the environment is associated with nature, rocks, and soil. In humans, the quality of earth is associated with structure, such as bone; it is also associated with an individual's sense of safety, security, boundaries and the emotions of fear and trust. A square is an earth shape and the musical note of 'C' carries the earth vibration (Stone 1987).

In order to understand how each element is represented in the body, the environment, and in life, it is important to first understand the qualities and attributes of each (Table 5.2). When exploring the characteristics of an element, it is important to be clear on your frame of reference. For example, a physical body, in and of itself, is an earth structure. Yet, when looking at different physical bodies you see shapes and sizes that correspond to the attributes

Table 5.2 An elemental look at the body (Frawley 1989, Burger 1998, Lad 1998, Svoboda 1989, Lloyd 2005)

Ether	Air	Fire	Water	Earth
Overall body – external factors	Psychological – mind	Psychological – emotions	Functional body	Structural body
Hair	Skin	Muscles	Flesh/fat	Bone
Head	Neck	Thorax	Waist	Lower limb
Thigh	Knee	Leg	Ankle	Foot
Upper Arm	Elbow	Lower Arm	Wrist	Hand
Big toe, thumb	2nd toe, index finger	3rd toe or finger	4th toe or ring finger	5th toe or finger
Distal phalanx	Distal interphalangeal joint	Middle phalanx	Proximal interphalangeal joint	Proximal phalanx

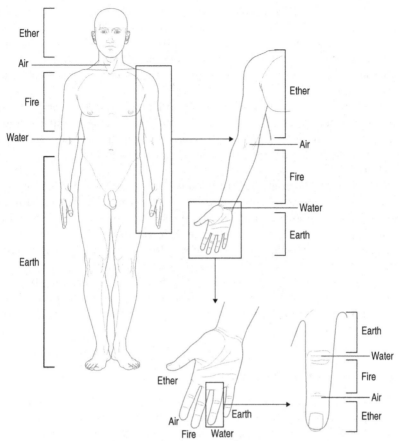

Fig 5.5 An elemental breakdown of the body. Notice how the ether aspects are the most proximal aspects of the body until you reach the hands and feet. At this point the energy waves return to source and the ether aspects are distal.

of each element. We can explore each part of the body in increasingly infinite detail, as shown below and in Fig. 5.5.

General characteristics of the elements

All elements come from *ether*. Ether encompasses the two extremes – an individual's personal essence, and their external environment. A person's essence is their core, their inner self, or blueprint. Ether is the place of inner spirituality, tranquility, and neutrality. A person's external environment is everything that is outside of the body. It consists of factors such as: where one lives, the seasons, the weather, an individual's work environment, their family and friends, the noise, sound, and light that they encounter on a daily basis. Ether patterns manifest in a person's vitality and their will to live. Ether is the presence of energy overall. It, in and of itself, doesn't have a definite form, but it is conveyed in the quality of all energy.

Air is the main element of movement. It represents the psychological aspect of the mind and expression of speech. It has the qualities of diversity, spontaneity, and speed. Air is light, dry, and flexible. The movement of the air element is primarily east to west around the body. It is associated with the nervous system and it regulates the electrical impulses in the body.

Fire is direction, force, power, time, and focus. It represents the psychological aspect of emotions. It has the quality of being impulsive, motivating, and exciting. It can also be overpowering, frustrating and angry. Fire is warming and drying in nature. The movement of fire is in a spiral direction.

Water, like air, is an element of movement. It is represented in the functional aspect of the body. It is the element of nurture, creativity, intuition, unconscious emotion, and adaptability. It can be cleansing and compassionate or very needy and compulsive. Water is moist and cooling in nature. The movement of water is flowing and it moves from cephalad to caudal, that is it moves between the north and south poles of the body.

Earth is the element of strength and form. It represents the structural aspect of the body and the sense of boundaries, safety and support. It has the qualities of routine, consistency, structure, and details. Earth is warm and drying in nature.

Ether quality of the elements

Table 5.3 shows the qualities of ether in nature and how it manifests in astrology, sound, food, and art. Understanding the ether aspect of the elements is a valuable tool to assist in a treatment strategy for a patient. For example, if you determine that the underlying root cause is a deficiency of earth, you can add earth foods to a patient's diet, or recommend that they take up sculpting, or listen to drumming.

Mental qualities of the elements

The mind has an air quality. When exploring the mind you can hear how the differences in how individuals think and speak reveal different elemental qualities of the mind (see Table 5.4).

Emotional qualities of the elements

Emotions have a fire quality, but when looking solely at emotions you can see how all the elements are represented (Table 5.5).

The elemental aspects of the functional body

The functional body is represented by the water element (Table 5.6). Within the functional body itself, every element is represented. To fully understand the elemental aspects of the functional body, you require a

Table 5.3 Ether aspect of the elements (Frawley 1989, Burger 1998, Lad 1998, Svoboda 1989, Lloyd 2005)

	Ether	Air	Fire	Water	Earth
Colour	Blue	Green	Yellow	Orange	Red
Quality	Sense of self, self esteem	Moderation, self regulation	Reality, self expression	Dependence, self care	Boundaries, self protection
Purpose	Blueprint	Formation	Action	Reaction	Manifestation
Characteristic	Subtlety and Space	Movement	Transformation and light	Fluidity, liquified and cohesion	Solid, density
Action	Speaking	Grasping	Direction of movement	Procreativity	Excreting
Type of energy	Etheric energy	Electrical energy	Thermogenic or radiant energy	Chemical energy	Mechanical or physical energy
Environment	Space	Gas	Heat	Liquid	Solid
Focus on	Achievement 'I am'	Appearance 'I want'	Power 'I care'	People 'I need'	Material 'I have'
Gunas	Sattva	Rajas	Sattva & rajas	Sattva & tamas	Tamas
Sound	Silence 'G', HAM	High pitched Fast 'F', YAM	Loud, staccato 'E', RAM	Smooth, flowing 'D', VAM	Low, deep, slow, droning 'C', LAM
Sense	Hearing	Touch	Sight	Taste	Smell
Gem	Moonstone	Emerald	Coral	Pearl	Ruby
Art	Music	Dance	Painting	Cooking	Sculpture and aromas
Astrology	None	Gemini, Libra, Aquarius	Aries, Leo, Sagittarius	Cancer, Scorpio, Pisces	Taurus, Virgo, Capricorn
Planet	Mercury	Venus	Mars	Jupiter	Saturn
Metal	Mercury	Copper	Iron	Tin	Lead
Business	Marketplace, purpose	Sales	Finance and operations	Marketing and merchandising	Product or service
Numerology	'5'	'4' & '6'	'2' & '8'	'3' & '7'	'1' & '9'
Food	Sprouts	Fruit, nuts, sour, 8–12 feet (3–4 m) above the ground	Grains, legumes, 2–6 feet (1.5–2 m) above the ground, bitter and hot	Melons, green vegetables, ground level to 2 feet (1.5 m), salty and cold	Root vegetables, sweet and hot

Symptom patterns

Table 5.4 Mental qualities of the elements (Frawley 1989, Burger 1998, Lad 1998, Svoboda 1989, Lloyd 2005)

	Ether	Air	Fire	Water	Earth
Overall	Stillness	Mental activity	Intelligence	Creativity	Structure
Quality	Tranquility, peace, neutrality	Many thoughts & ideas, thinks before acting	Enthusiastic, willful, focused, perceptive	Sensitive, patient, fluid	Steady, enduring, routine
Attributes	Universal love, spaciousness & harmony	Attention, honesty & thought	Insight, power, quickness, motivated, inspirational	Intuition, receptivity, nurturing	Support, stability, practical, discrimination, slow & steady

Table 5.5 Emotional qualities of the elements (Frawley 1989, Burger 1998, Lad 1998, Svoboda 1989, Lloyd 2005)

	Ether	Air	Fire	Water	Earth
Overall	Freedom of expression	Gentleness	Warmth	Nurturing	Secure
Governs	Openness, inner self, expression	Lightness, diversity & movement	Sense of power, motivating	Adaptability & cleansing	Safety, basic existence & survival
Balanced	Identity, humble, pride	Honest, integrity & charity	Enthusiastic, forgiving, courage	Receptive compassionate	Protective, supporting
Yang	Arrogant, shameless	Impatient, illusions	Resentful, judging, anger	Compulsive, passionate, lust	Invulnerable, defensive, paranoid
Yin	Worthless, shamed, grief	Jealous, hopeless, desire	Controlled by others, frustration, competitive	Dependency, needy, attachment	No boundaries, anxious, fear

solid foundation in the qualities of the elements and in the physiology of the body.

The elemental aspects of the structural body

The structural body represents the earth quality of a person (Table 5.7). The different shapes and forms of the structural body are indicative of their elemental makeup.

Table 5.6 Elemental aspects of the functional body (Frawley 1989, Burger 1998, Lad 1998, Svoboda 1989, Lloyd 2005)

	Ether	Air	Fire	Water	Earth
Overall	Lengthening	Speed of response	Shaking	Flowing Movement	Contraction
Governs	Sleep	Thirst	Hunger	Luster	Laziness
Organs	Space	Chest cavity, lungs	Stomach, liver, spleen, heart, gallbladder	Bladder, secretory glands	Bone, colon & kidneys
Glands	Thyroid	Thymus	Pancreas	Ovaries & testis	Adrenals
Tissues	Cavities	Nerves	Ligaments, muscles	Fat, menstrual tissue	Blood, tendons
Fluid	Ovum, semen, CSF	Tears, breath	Enzymes, hormones	Lymph, plasma, sweat	Blood
Body systems	Joints, spinal column	Nervous system, circulation & respiration	Digestion, metabolism	Endocrine, lymphatic & reproductive	Skeletal, elimination & immune

CSF, cerebrospinal fluid.

Table 5.7 Elemental aspects of the structural body (Frawley 1989, Burger 1998, Lad 1998, Svoboda 1989, Lloyd 2005)

	Ether	Air	Fire	Water	Earth
Overall	Hair	Skin	Muscles	Flesh/fat	Bone
Positive pole	Head/ears	Shoulders/lungs	Eyes, forehead	Chest, breast	Neck
Neutral pole	Sacrum	Kidneys	Solar plexus	Pelvis	Colon
Negative pole	Arch of foot	Ankles/calves	Thighs	Feet	Knees
Body type	Overall appearance	Light, thin, wiry & underweight	Moderate, lean & muscular	Moderate to stout, padded look, easy to gain weight	Moderate to heavy build, square, firm structure
Chakra	Throat	Heart	Solar plexus	Sacral	Root

QUALITIES OF SPECIFIC SYMPTOMS

The body has a limited way of expressing imbalances and disharmony. The same symptom can occur for a number of different reasons and determining a treatment strategy that is beneficial for the patient is dependent on being able to decipher what the symptoms are trying to convey. The specific qualities and characteristics of each symptom reveal their underlying pattern. This pattern will relate back to the causal factors. The following provides a look at how common symptoms can be assessed according to the qualities and characteristics that they manifest.

Pain

Pain is a complex physiological and psychological phenomenon. It is an alarm sign of the body that something is wrong and it can originate from misalignment, from congestion, from a state of excess or deficiency. It can arise from disharmony in bone, organs, tissues, or vessels. It is an important symptom and is best not to suppress. Overall pain is an air quality, as air is the element that governs the nervous system and the nervous system governs all sensations (Lad 2005). The specific qualities of pain are highly subjective and variable, and they are influenced by many factors, these other factors bringing in the qualities of the other elements. For example:

- *Air pain* is variable, migrating, throbbing, and cutting. It is better heat and worse cold. The area of pain is dry, scaly, or cracked.
- *Fire pain* is hot or has a burning sensation. It is better cold and worse hot and is usually better after rest. The area is red and inflamed, and there is often sweating. The site of the pain might be irritating, and frustrating to the patient.
- *Water pain* involves swelling and edema. The skin is often oily and moist, especially when there is an excess of water. The pain is better with heat and worse with cold. The pain is often aggravated in damp weather.
- *Earth pain* creates a sense of heaviness, a dull ache. The pain is often localized and can involve congestion in the area or an erosion of the tissues or structures. The pain is usually better with movement and worse after resting.

Fatigue

Fatigue is an indication of decreased energy and is associated with many different diseases, especially chronic diseases, degenerative diseases, and diseases that are hard to treat (Frawley 1989, Seller 2000). Fatigue can be due to an acute healing response, a reaction to the current stressors of life, poor lifestyle habits, or it can be chronic. Chronic fatigue is a deficiency pattern that can be associated with any element, and typically is associated with them all. The energy of the body comes from different sources: a patient's constitution and from food and breath. It is also affected by a patient's mental activity and their lifestyle. When fatigue is a primary concern for a patient, the role of the practitioner is to determine as many factors as possible that are contributing and to provide a treatment strategy that is building and nourishing to the patient. As digestion requires a lot of energy, and as it is a common cause or aggravating factor, the treatment of fatigue often starts by addressing a patient's diet and their digestive fire.

Constipation

Constipation results from food and water imbalances, inhibition of the muscular contraction of the bowels, obstruction to the bowels, or it can be due to imbalances in the digestive or nervous system. An old-time naturopathic belief was that 'disease begins in the colon' (Pizzorno & Murray 2000). The bowels are an organ of elimination which makes them an earth organ. The following clarify the role of the other elements.

Air governs the nervous system which is responsible for the contraction of the musculature of the bowels. Constipation due to an air pattern has the quality of small, rabbit-pellet like stools accompanied by a lot of gas and abdominal distention. The air element is also the element of the mind and constipation is often caused by increased mental activity, worry and anxiety, over stimulation of the nervous system; in other words a patient's energy is in their head versus in their bowels. The consumption of air food – dry or light food – can also be a contributing factor (Frawley 1989).

Fire governs the overall digestive function. Constipation can be caused by a weakness in digestive fire, fever, or excess internal heat.

Water governs the body fluids. Constipation can be caused by a decrease in body fluids, or body fluids that are too viscous. Food and eating are nourishing to the body, and nourishing is a water characteristic. When the consumption of food is imbalanced, either in excess, deficient, or incongruent with a person's constitution, it can impact the bowels. For example, certain foods, such as dairy and bananas are constipating for many people. Eating too quickly or eating when anxious or upset also are factors.

Earth governs the structure of the bowel wall. Obstruction, polyps, masses, etc. involve an imbalance in the earth element.

Fever

Fever is a defense measure of the body against disease and as such is typically a curative reaction (Vogel 1959). If a fever is suppressed the disease, unopposed by the fever, gets stronger. A fever is an adaptation response of the body to an infection, but it can also be caused by other factors and at times a patient may feel feverish, yet there is no rise in body temperature. Fever is an internal increase of heat. This feeling of heat might be in response to 'fire' emotions such as anger, irritability, frustration, jealousy, or fear. The emotion that is attached with the fever will guide a practitioner to the elemental quality.

Internal fever creates canker sores, fever blisters, or aches and pains. Mental fever can be due to incompatible food combining, wrong lifestyle and diet, and the application of extremes of hot and cold (Lad 2005).

Air fever is associated with shivering, body ache that tends to wander, constipation, and nervous system symptoms, such as tinnitus. The temperature is not that high and the fever often creates insomnia and anxiety.

Fire fever is associated with high temperatures, hot flashes and flushed skin, and a sense of nausea and vomiting. The urine is often dark yellow and the pulses are rapid.

Water fever is associated with sweating and pale skin, runny nose, and a feeling of cold and congestion.

SYMBOLISM OF BODY PARTS

Every body part has a physical function, a purpose, and an energetic meaning, both literal and figurative. The physical function and purpose provide insight into the energetic meaning. The more you understand what you do with the different aspects of your body and how disharmony in that body part affects you, the easier it is to correlate it with the energetics. Yet, the reason why the body shifts in a particular fashion for one person often is different for someone else. It depends on a person's constitution, their susceptibility, their life experiences, and the root cause of the energetic shift. For example, for some, a painful shoulder represents the inability to work, for others it is the inability to hug someone they love, for someone else it means the loss of independence because they cannot drive, or it indicates that they are tired of carrying a lot of responsibility, and for yet another, it is a message to slow down and to be more careful. What is common is that a person's ability to give and receive, or to push and pull, has been affected. As a practitioner it is advisable to have a general sense of the energetics of each aspect and then listen to how a patient relays their history. The specifics will be unique for each individual, but there will be a similarity and uniqueness to the symbolism for each aspect of the body.

There are functional, structural, and psychological attributes to each part of the body. For example, the structural purpose of the back is to give the body form, structure, and posture; the functional purpose is about motion and it provides a channel for nerves; psychologically the back stands for support, the past, and a feeling of strength. When there is a specific body part that is susceptible, understand the structural, functional, and psychological purpose, and then see how these purposes correlate to the patient's 'story'.

As you explore the following symbolism of specific body parts, keep an open mind. Look for as many explanations and purposes for each part. It is the subtleties, not the generalities that make them applicable. The generalities point a practitioner in a specific direction; they start the conversation, which only the patient is able to finish. For example, a patient may have recurring weakness in their left ankle that is not associated with a physical injury. The left is the Yin side of the body, which represents the characteristics such as, nourishment, creativity, rest, receiving from others. The ankle is a water joint which means it relates to flowing movement, compassion, relationships. The purpose of the ankle is assist with balance and groundedness. Its function is to support walking, or moving forward. Listen to see if any aspect of the patient's story conveys these same themes, especially a lack of these qualities, based on the fact that the ankle is weak. The following are some general guidelines for the energetics of the body:

• The midline or centre of the body relates to one's self, core issues, and one's beliefs.

- The extremities relate more to our interaction with the external environment and the impact of other people or situations.
- The intensity of the shift is either a reflection of the depth of the energetic impact or the need to change.

Examples of body symbolism

- The purpose of the arms is to give and receive. They involve taking what you desire or deserve from life, pushing forward or pulling back.
- The purpose of hands is grasping and letting go, touching and feeling.
- Legs are for moving forward or backwards, going towards something that you desire and look forward to, or moving away from something. The meaning is about having the direction and sense of ability to move into the next phase of your life or in a different direction.
- Feet have to do with how you step into your life. They have to do with balance and groundedness and they represent the chronic aspect of our energy patterns.
- The back represents motion. It is the motor aspect of the body. It also represents the past. It provides support and strength. It provides the structure and posture to the body.
- The front is the sensory aspect of the body. All the senses are located on the front. It is the acute or present aspect of health. The front provides the look and feel of a person. Most people view themselves primarily on how the front of their body looks.
- The chest is about openness to the outside world. The chest cavity houses the lungs and heart, two organs associated with love and sadness. The chest represents comfort with expression.

ASSESSMENT CONCEPTS AND ANALOGIES

The following naturopathic medical concepts provide practitioners with a framework for communicating the concepts of health and disease to patients. Analogies are valuable as they allow detailed concepts to be understood more simply.

The waves of health and disease

Human beings are complex organisms comprised of vibrating energy fields. Every part; every organ, cell, tissue, and molecule has its own energy field and wave pattern.

A useful analogy between simple and complex forms is the difference between plucking a single string (which represents a simple organism like an amoeba) and playing an entire orchestra (which represents a complex organism like a human being) (Sylver 2008).

When an individual is in a healthy state, the wave patterns are organized and in sync; when unhealthy the waves are disorganized and out of sync. A 'symphony' when all is well; a 'cacophony' when all is not well. Every cell in the body is a transmitter and receiver for different wave patterns. As a practitioner you can listen, palpate, and measure these different wave patterns as a means of assessing health. The most common waves that are assessed are the pulse, respiration, movement of muscles, and cranial rhythm; yet even emotions and thoughts can be thought of as a wave. The difference between health and disease lies in the relative freedom of movement between every part (Sills 1989). For example, a healthy blood pressure of 120/80 has particular wave pattern to it, as noted in the range between the systolic and diastolic measurements. When the range between the systolic and diastolic becomes too wide or too narrow, or the overall readings go too high or too low, it indicates a health problem (Beers & Berkow 1999).

Every wave pattern has a normal amplitude and frequency range, with set upper and lower limits. In a normal wave pattern, there is the ability to adapt and compensate more easily to external and internal changes. For example, heart rate variability (HRV) measures the variations in heart rate and the autonomic regulation of circulatory function. Research has shown that when the HRV wave pattern is maximized an individual's tolerance of stress increases, their perception of pain decreases, respiration improves, and sleep and mood improves (Hassett et al 2007). When assessing a patient's breath, you expect the movement on the right and left sides of the ribs to be symmetrical and the breathing pattern to be normal (Chaitow et al 2002).

When in a state of overwhelm, the frequency, amplitude, or wave patterns change; indicating that an individual is less healthy, it is not as strong, flexible, or tolerant, and is not able to adjust with the same ease. At times, the wave pattern is still in the normal range and has a normal wave pattern, yet the amplitude has decreased and the frequency has increased; see wave pattern (b) in Fig 5.6. When disease sets in the wave pattern becomes disorganizes and erratic, and it also might shift above or below the normal range; see wave pattern (c) in Fig. 5.6.

Layers of life

The experiences of life can be viewed as layers (Fig. 5.7). Each layer represents a different event or situation that has had an impact. Some layers strengthen health and others detract from it. The center represents a person's constitution, the strengths and weaknesses that they were born with. The most superficial layer represents present time.

The layers represent psychological, functional, and structural events and changes. Positive situations and healthy lifestyles support health and create layers of strength. Situations or lifestyle factors that detract from health create layers that contract a person's energy, resulting in decreased health and vitality. The state of health, at any point in time, is a reflection of the accumulation of the layers.

During life there often is a common thread or theme to the events that have impacted health. For example, a patient repeatedly encounters situations where they were taken advantage of, or where they didn't feel good enough, or they will frequently have respiratory or digestive flare-ups.

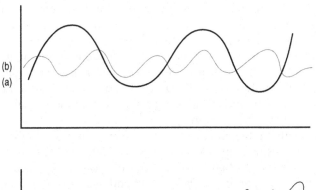

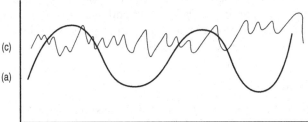

Fig 5.6 Waves of health and disease. (a) Health – organized wave pattern, with 'normal' amplitude and frequency. (b) State of overwhelm – organized wave pattern, with shortened amplitude and increased frequency. (c) Disease – disorganized wave pattern, wave outside of normal range.

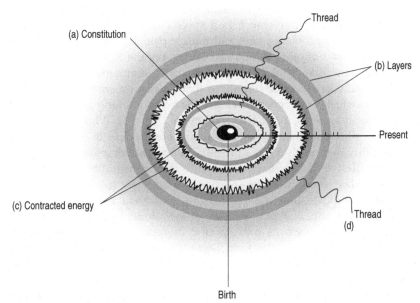

Fig 5.7 Layers of life. From Lloyd 2005, with permission from the author. (a) Constitution – reflects the qualities and attributes that a person was born with. (b) Layers – the significant events and situations build on each other. Positive events and situations strengthen or add to our health and result in an expansion of energy. (c) Contracted energy – occurs in response to events or situations that are still unresolved and have a negative impact on health. (d) Threads – represent common factors that have disrupted health over time and that continue to play a disruptive role.

Through the healing process, you can address many layers that are detracting from health at once when you treat the root cause of the energetic thread. For example, if a patient has a history of being overly fearful and cautious, this emotion will affect many aspects or situations throughout their life. When the root cause of the fear is addressed, it decreases the negative impact of all the layers involved. If the thread relates to an imbalance in lifestyle factors, correcting these often significantly improves an individual's quality of life and eases the overall healing process.

Healing begins at the outer layer. That means, starting with the symptoms that occurred most recently. As one layer is addressed, the symptoms of the underlying layer will often become more noticeable. For each level there are initiating and aggravating factors. By addressing common aggravating factors, and treating the outermost layers in sequence, the healing process for a patient is more gentle and effective.

Plate of symptoms

It is rare for a patient to present with only one symptom. Often there are a number of symptoms that can be grouped together by the timing of their onset and the organ system or systems that they correspond to. For example, a patient might have had a few of the symptoms their whole life; some might have started 10 years ago, some 2 years ago, and then others more recently. This indicates that there are at least four symptom patterns or layers occurring simultaneously.

Signs and symptoms that started concurrently often convey the same pattern and they are due to the same initiating and aggravating factors. For example, having intolerance to a specific food can result in digestive complaints, sinus problems, joint and muscle pain, bloating, fatigue, insomnia and a number of other symptoms. The role of the naturopathic doctor is to find the pattern and link between the various symptoms.

When you take all of the symptoms that a patient reports and map them on a circle, which has concentric rings representing timing and slices representing organ systems, a pattern will emerge (Fig. 5.8). When a patient has been struggling with symptoms their whole life it points to a constitutional susceptibility that needs to be addressed by the patient understanding how to choose lifestyle habits that are suited to their constitution. Symptoms in a specific slice – organ system – that started later in life and are still continuing, indicate that the initiating factors were never appropriately addressed. If a patient lists a number of symptoms indicating imbalances in both systemic functions and specific organs, it is helpful to address the building blocks to health first. Doing so often will 'clear the plate' of a number of symptoms and assist in identifying the symptoms that have a deeper root cause.

When you look at an array of symptoms that are occurring in a number of organs or systems an energetic pattern often emerges. The following examples illustrate manifestations of imbalances in earth – a history of broken bones, prolapsed bladder, feeling of not being supported or strong enough to deal with the challenges in life indicate a deficiency of earth in the core,

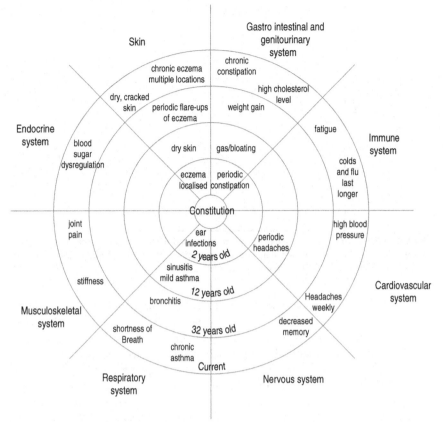

Fig 5.8 Plate of symptoms.

while chronic stiffness and calcification of joints indicate an excess of earth in the periphery. Symptoms either display an imbalance in one or more of the elements, or will display a disharmonic balancing between elements. For example, an excess of fire can result in a deficiency of water – the fire has 'burned off' the water.

Wellness delta

Wellness ranges from optimal health to debilitating disease. The delta or span between these two points is an indication of an individual's state of wellness and health (Fig. 5.9). When the delta is large, a person 'has a lot of room to play' and can withstand a lot of stress and disharmony prior to showing signs of disease; when the delta is small, an individual's resistance is low and they more easily succumb to disease. Where an individual 'sits' on the path between a healthy state and one of disease, the delta between is a reflection of their constitution as well as the accumulation of their experiences.

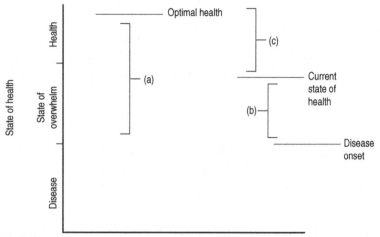

Fig 5.9 Wellness delta. (a) Wide delta between health and onset of symptoms or disease. (b) Narrow delta between current state and the onset of symptoms or disease. (c) Difference between current state of health and optimal health.

Each organ system or aspect of the body also has a specific susceptibility. The greater the susceptibility of an organ system, the smaller the delta between health and disease, and hence the greater the need to be aware of factors that disrupt health. For example, if a patient has a susceptible digestive system then they will react to specific food or quantities of food, more so than a patient who has a strong digestive system. For the patient with the weaker system, it is more imperative to address digestive factors, such as quality and quantity of food, relationship between food and stress, importance of regular bowel movements, etc.

Factors that disrupt health and are not resolved have a cumulative effect, and over time decrease the span of the delta. For example, a patient with anxiety might find that their anxiety is worse with the consumption of sugar, alcohol, caffeine; with dehydration; with decreased activity and increased time spent on the computer; with decreased sleep and a disrupted routine; and when stressful situations occur. The initial aim of treatment is to address those factors that you have control over – diet, exercise, water, lifestyle routine, and breathing, with the expectation that doing so increases the delta and provides a greater 'buffer' for handling stressful situations that you have less control over.

REFERENCES

Beers MH, Berkow R 1999 The Merck Manual of Diagnosis and Therapy, Seventeenth Edition. Merck Research Laboratories, New Jersey

Beinfield H, Korngold E 1991 Between Heaven and Earth, a Guide to Chinese Medicine. Ballantine Publishing, New York

Burger B 1998 Esoteric Anatomy, the Body as Consciousness. North Atlantic Books, California

Chaitow L, Bradley D, Gilbert C 2002 Multidisciplinary Approaches to Breathing Pattern Disorders. Churchill Livingstone, Edinburgh

Frawley D 1989 Ayurvedic Healing, a Comprehensive Guide. Passage Press, Utah

Hassett AL, Radvanski DC, Vaschillo EG, et al 2007 A pilot study of the efficacy of heart rate variability (HRV) biofeedback in patients with fibromyalgia. Appl Psychophyiol Biofeedback 32:1–10

Kaptchuk TJ 1983 The Web That Has No Weaver, Understanding Chinese Medicine. Congdon & Weed, Chicago

Lad V 1998 Ayurveda, the Science of Self-healing. Motilal Banarsidass Publishers. Delhi

Lad V 2005 Ayurvedic Perspectives on Selected Pathologies. The Ayurvedic Press, New Mexico

Lloyd IR 2005 Messages from the Body, a Guide to the Energetics Of Health. Naturopathic Publications, Toronto

Maciocia G 1989 The Foundations of Chinese Medicine, a Comprehensive Text for Acupuncturists and Herbalists. Churchill Livingstone, Edinburgh

Maciocia G 1998 The Foundations of Chinese Medicine. Churchill Livingstone, Edinburgh

Pizzorno JE, Murray MT 2000 Textbook of Natural Medicine, volume I & II, second edition. Churchill Livingstone, Edinburgh

Seller RH 2000 Differential Diagnosis of Common Complaints, fourth edition. WB Saunders, Philadelphia

Sills F 1989 The Polarity Process, Energy as a Healing Art. Element Books, Dorset

Stone R 1987 Polarity Therapy, volume two. CRCS Publications, California

Svoboda RE 1989 Prakruit, Your Ayurvedic constitution. Geocom, New Mexico

Sylver N, 2008 Healing with Electromedicine and Sound Therapies, part one. Townsend Letter, February/March:93–99

Vogel A 1959 The Nature Doctor. Bioforce-Verlag, Switzerland

FURTHER READING

Bridges L 2004 Face Reading in Chinese Medicine. Churchill Livingstone, Missouri

Collins RD 1997 Differential Diagnosis of Common Complaints, fourth edition. WB Saunders, Philadelphia

Hammer LI 2005 Chinese Pulse Diagnosis, a Contemporary Approach, revised edition. Eastland Press, Seattle

Isenberg N, Silbersweing D, Engelian A, et al 1999 Linguistic threat activates the human amygdala. Proc Natl Acad Sci USA, 96(18):10456–10459

Knaster M 1996 Discovering the Body's Wisdom. Bantam Books, New York

Lu HC 1994 Chinese Natural Cures, Traditional Methods for Remedies and Preventions. Black Dog & Leventhal Publishing, New York

Monte T 1991 Reading the Body, Ohashi's Book of Oriental Diagnosis. Penguin Books, New York

Morningstar A 2001 The Ayurvedic Guide to Polarity Therapy: Hands on Healing. Lotus Press, Wisconsin

Pert C 2002 The Wisdom of the Receptors: Neuropeptides, the Emotions, and Bodymind. Advances 18(1):30–35

Pole S 2006 Ayurvedic Medicine, the Principles of Traditional Practice. Elsevier, Philadelphia

Rossi E 2007 Shen, Psycho-Emotional Aspects of Chinese Medicine. Elsevier, China

Sagar SM 2001 Restored Harmony, An Evidence Based Approach for Integrating Traditional Chinese Medicine into Complementary Cancer Care. Dreaming Dragon Fly Communications, Hamilton

Stone R 1985 Health Building. CRCS Wellness Books, Tennessee

Stone R 1986 Polarity Therapy, volume one. CRCS Publications, California

CHAPTER 6
Causes of symptoms and diseases

Human beings are complex systems that are able to adjust to a tremendous amount of internal and external stimuli while still maintaining a homeody-namic state. Symptoms and disease arise when a patient is overwhelmed or exhausted and is no longer able to adapt and compensate to disrupting factors. The onset of signs and symptoms themselves can be a positive message; it simply indicates a need for something to be addressed or changed. The breadth of the assessment, and the perspective and beliefs that a practitioner attaches to signs and symptoms influences the outcome and the direction that a practitioner will follow.

> Wholistic medicine focuses on body, emotions, mind, relationships and spirit. This extends the range of conceptualization of the causes of illnesses and of potential ways for dealing with them (Benor 2006).

The conventional medical system has a different model. For example, a book on differential diagnosis states, 'the causes of each symptom can be analyzed by one or more of the basic sciences of anatomy, histology, physiology, and biochemistry' (Collins 1997). Only the tangible components of the body are included, with the omission of all environmental and exter-nal factors, let alone lifestyle, the intangible, or the spiritual. In the field of naturopathic medicine, assessing the cause of symptoms and disease involves understanding the factors that initiated the state of overwhelm, not just the overt manifestation of overwhelm.

THE NATUROPATHIC PERSPECTIVE

The naturopathic perspective is that health and disease is logical; there is a meaning and purpose behind symptoms and disease states. This perspective is similar to Chinese medicine where the belief is that the continual overuse and depletion of the inherited Qi or life force is the cause of disease (Bridges 2004). Every patient requires specific internal and external nutrients, substances and qualities – such as love and a purpose to live – to function and survive. If these are not present, or they are present in excess, then they can result in a disruption in health.

Not all diseases are the result of wrong-doing, or wrong-thinking. The health and disease of human beings is interrelated to the health of the environment, external factors, their community, and to nature itself. Naturo-pathic medicine recognizes that there is a higher power or spiritual force that controls life and at times 'bad' things happen for reasons that we can't always understand in the present moment. Yet most diseases, especially chronic diseases, are largely a result of cumulative effects on a patient's life. Recognizing and acknowledging that health and disease follow certain laws is essential to understanding the patterns of health and disease that continu-ously emerge. The belief that disease is random, and that it can happen to anyone at any time, is a characteristic of the current fear-based conventional medical system. This erroneous belief separates patients from their lifestyle and from their environment; it takes away personal responsibility and envi-ronmental responsibility. It puts the emphasis of medical research on treat-ment instead of prevention, and on drugs and interventions instead of lifestyle education and self-responsibility. It is unrealistic and arrogant to think, or to base a medical system, on the delusion that the most complex living systems, humans, are the only living systems that do not follow the laws of Nature. What is realistic is that human beings are complex systems that are integrated and inseparable from their environment, lifestyle, family, and community. We might not fully understand all the laws of Nature, or life, but there is a difference between knowing how everything works versus believing and looking for the logic as to how everything works. For example, there was the recognition that a patient's thoughts affected their health long before there was an understanding of how it actually happens.

Recognizing that health and disease happen for a reason does not put it in the realm of linear causality. You cannot always say that one factor alone causes disease. Human beings are complex systems, with multiple components and levels of complexity and susceptibility. For example, one belief is that germs cause disease and if exposed you are likely to get sick. The naturopathic perspective recognizes the 'disease-carrying' feature of germs, but puts the emphasis of whether or not a patient gets sick on their resistance and susceptibility. The germ is a variable, but the strength of a patient's vitality, their current level of health, their current adherence to a healthy lifestyle, and their overall susceptibility has as much or more of a bearing than the germ itself; hence, the emphasis of whether or not a patient gets sick is mostly under their control, not an external factor. Human beings are complex systems and as such, their thinking is contextual; it is based on the mutual relationship between the variables and the specific nuances and considerations of each specific time and place. The aim, during any assessment process, is to determine the variables that are at play for each patient, and to what degree they are a contributing factor to the disease state.

The task of uncovering the variables that are impacting a patient's health often is daunting due to the unlimited number of these variables and the constant increase in number of factors. One hundred years ago, even 50 years ago, the number of factors that impacted health was different; it was simpler. The introduction of vaccinations, chemicals in patient care products, plastics, fillers and additives in food, substances used in dental procedures, cell phones, computers, pesticides and insecticides, the impact of manufacturing, mining, pollution, surgery, implants, and so on, has greatly increased the factors and variables that need to be considered in order to thoroughly assess any symptom or disease state.

Although the overall number of variables is unlimited, it is limited for each patient. The purpose of an intake is to determine the breadth of factors that need to be considered. The family and lifestyle history, and the pattern of onset of symptoms, in itself, assists in focusing the assessment in a specific direction. For example, smoking is a factor, but only if a patient smokes or if they are around people who smoke. In order for a variable to be a factor, a patient needs to have had exposure. For example, to narrow the possible number of factors due to the environment, a practitioner would ask a patient about where they were born, where they grew up, how they spent their time, the age and type of house they lived in and how it was heated, the presence of factories or industry or hydro towers around them, etc. The practitioner would then take the patient's input and correlate it with the factors that are known about an area; for example, if a patient grew up in an area where there had been mining, then heavy metal toxicity would be a consideration in the assessment. Each disease and symptom also has a number of variables that are known to be considerations. It is possible, and often valuable, to work backwards based on a patient's presenting symptoms to expand the assessment variables.

Health and disease is a two-way continuum. Whether the body is heading toward health or disease depends on the 'mode' that the body is in. When the initiating factors are addressed and the body is in the mode of healing, it will heal itself provided it has the needed building blocks. On the other hand, when the symptoms are being ignored or suppressed, and the wisdom of the body is being over-ridden with drugs, surgery, or treatments that mask the symptoms, a patient might remain on a path progressing towards disease. For example, if a patient, a couple months after her daughter is killed in a car accident, is diagnosed with a breast cyst that 'looks suspicious', the initiating factor – the reason her body went into shock – might be the news of her daughter's death. Having the cyst removed without addressing the psychological state does not address the root cause. In this case the mode of the patient will probably still be 'on the path' to disease. It is not a question of whether removing the cyst is appropriate or not; that depends on the mindset of the patient. What matters is whether or not the root cause is addressed. Simply removing the cyst might mean that a patient 'holds the trauma' in another, often deeper, part of the body.

It is not difficult to impose *change* on the body; the body is energy after all and will respond to any energetic influence that it comes in contact with. What is difficult is having the body maintain a healthy change on a cellular and energetic level. The introduction of natural or conventional therapeutics might slow down, prolong, or lessen the burden on the body but they won't create a shift to health that holds if the body is still being triggered on some level. For change to be held, the initiating factors of disease have to be addressed.

FACTORS TO CONSIDER

When assessing the causes of symptoms and diseases it is important to look at the initiating factors, the aggravating factors and the ameliovating factors.

Initiating factors

Initiating factors cause a state of overwhelm, shock, or energetic shift. They are the root causes of symptoms and diseases. When the onset of symptoms are sudden, the initiating factor is usually an event or situation that occurred, such as an accident, a traumatic situation like being embarrassed in public for the first time, being fired, or hearing that a loved one has died, or a situation such as food poisoning, or an allergic reaction. When the onset of the symptoms is gradual, the initiating factor is usually an imbalance in the building blocks to health or chronic exposure to an external disrupting factor, like heavy metals or cigarette smoke.

Initiating factors often need to be addressed and resolved in order for the body to heal. These factors, especially when due to a specific situation, continue to signal the body that it is in a state of disharmony, that there is a problem.

Addressing these initiating factors breaks the cycle or pattern of disease and allows the signal to 'turn off'. A patient can then return to the mode of healing.

Symptoms associated with initiating factors relate to the primary site of manifestation. The primary site of manifestation is not necessarily the site with the most severe or the most notable symptoms; it is the site that is linked most closely to the factor or factors that initiated the shift away from health. The role of the naturopathic doctor is to identify the initiating factors, to address the root cause of disease, to remove the obstacles to cure, and in doing so, to stimulate the healing power of the body.

Aggravating factors

Aggravating factors intensify, minimize, or alter signs and symptoms, and they weaken a patient's strength and healing potential. For example, consuming multiple cups of coffee a day might minimize the symptoms of fatigue, but it also aggravates the symptoms of insomnia. A patient's constitution dictates the factors that are most likely to be aggravating. For example, a patient who has a 'cold' constitution will be aggravated in the winter, with cold food or by drinking cold drinks.

Often aggravating factors are considered 'obstacles to cure' as they maintain or intensify the state of overwhelm, preventing a patient from healing completely. These factors are typically due to deficiencies and excesses in the building blocks, or they are due to environmental and external factors. For example, a patient might be more short-tempered if they haven't had sufficient sleep. They might find that their digestion is poor when they are angry as they tend to hold in their anger. A patient might find that when they eat any of the nightshade vegetables it affects a joint that was injured in the past. A patient tends to have recurring back pain due to poor ergonomics at work. A patient might find that consuming sugar intensifies their anxiety or blood sugar. There are many different factors that aggravate a patient. In many situations, it is helpful to improve the building blocks to health and to address the obvious external factors first, thus 'clearing the plate' of symptoms and making it easier to determine if there is an unresolved deeper factor.

> *In any given challenge to homeostasis, the ecology of the body is improved by reducing the number of factors which strain the resources that enable the body to heal itself (Mitchell 2007).*

Ameliorating factors

Ameliorating factors decrease or alleviate the intensity or onset of symptoms. The factors that ameliorate symptoms often provide a guide as to what has caused the aggravation. For example, a patient might not realize that they have a headache when they do not eat, but what they do realize is that their headache goes away when they do eat. The factors that ameliorate symptoms often balance the excesses or deficiencies of the aggravating factors, or balance the constitutional state of a patient. Having patients increase their awareness of the correlation between their lifestyle and their symptoms is an important aspect of self-care.

Associated signs and symptoms

Associated signs and symptoms might hold a closer connection to the initiating and aggravating factors than the primary symptom that a patient is concerned about. For example, a patient may present with hypertension which in and of itself, does not indicate the initiating and aggravating factors. In this case, the associated signs and symptoms will provide a better guide as to the causal factors and will be a better measurement of the resolution or progression of the concern. For example, hypertension can be associated with increased toxins in the colon, with psychological stress, excesses or imbalance in diet, with urinary problems, etc. The overall effect on the body is a constriction of vessels, an increase in viscosity of fluids, or a deposition of fat particle narrowing the arteries (Lad 2005). The symptom pattern of associated signs and symptoms leads a practitioner to determine the initiating and aggravating factors.

NATURE OF SYMPTOMS

There is seldom one single factor or cause for a disease state. Typically, there are a number of factors and variables with varying degrees of impact. How and where the symptoms associated with the disease manifest, how they correlate to a patient's constitution, lifestyle, environment, and the characteristics of the signs and symptoms, guide a practitioner to uncover the factors that caused the disruption in health. The nature of symptoms, such as the onset, intensity, and frequency provide key subjective information that assist in isolating the specific initiating and aggravating factors. They also relate to the patient's experience of their symptoms and the impact that their symptoms are having on their life. The aim of the practitioner is to correlate the patient's subjective experience of symptoms with the factors that caused them, and then, to look at the objective physical findings and laboratory tests to determine the degree to which the factors have disrupted the homeodynamic state.

Prior to understanding the nature of symptoms, it is important to recognize those factors that might be distorting the normal response of the body. For example, prescription medication, supplements, and even some treatments might alter the true expression of bodily symptoms. The more a patient is medicated, the more likely the true symptoms are being suppressed and overridden. In this situation, the symptoms are more likely to be an indication of how the body is responding to medication or treatment; not necessarily a reflection of how a patient is responding to the factors that disrupted health.

Understanding the characteristics or nature of symptoms requires an in-depth knowledge of anatomy, physiology, pathology, and the medical sciences, as well as an understanding of the mechanism of action of drugs and supplements, and the impact of other forms of treatment. It requires an appreciation and recognition of the body as a complex holistic system that is energetic, integrated and changing all the time. Symptoms are a wonderful diagnostic road map that can be interpreted by a skilled practitioner. A skilled practitioner also recognizes that there is not always a direct correlation between the discomfort that a patient is experiencing and the degree of risk to health. For example, the presence of pain might be very distressing to a patient and dramatically impact their quality of life, but it doesn't necessarily mean that their health concerns are of high risk.

Onset

The onset is about *when* signs and symptoms started. The strength of a patient's constitution, their susceptibilities, and the type and severity of the impact all influence *when* signs and symptoms start to appear.

The dimension which contributes most to the organization and clarity of the history is chronology. Dates and times serve to anchor the history in such a way that relationships between symptoms and events can be more clearly seen (Morgan & Engel 1969).

The shift from homeodynamic state can be thought of as a process due to a sudden insult, a gradual insult or progressive insult.

- The *sudden* onset of symptoms typically occurs directly after a significant situation; for example, a fall, a car accident, a heart attack, a natural disaster, an emotional shock, or a stressful situation. Whenever a patient links the onset of symptoms with a specific date, event, or situation, then something about that event has likely contributed to the state of overwhelm. The sudden onset of symptoms can also indicate an acute healing response, such as a fever at the onset of flu, or vomiting and diarrhea after eating bad food, or a skin reaction to a food that a patient has a high IgE hypersensitivity reaction to. When the onset is sudden, the body goes into a state of overwhelm and there is a dramatic shift or change in some aspect which alerts a patient to the need to pay attention, to change, to react or to take notice. There are times when a sudden event, such as a heart attack, is due to dissipative lifestyle (excessive consumption of food and drink, stressful work, sedentary lifestyle, poor sleep habits) and then a seemingly small situation becomes 'the straw that broke the camel's back.'
- The onset of *gradual* symptoms is due to a prolonged state of deficiency or excess, or due to chronic exposure to disruptive environmental or external factors. In these cases, the changes occur more subtly; as the body becomes weakened, exhausted, or less functional over time. Gradual changes are a result of an imbalance between what you take in and what you eliminate; what you need and what you take in. The constant state of imbalance and overwhelm results in decreased innate healing, increased susceptibility and adds to the progression of disease. There isn't a direct cause and effect because of the time lag and the numerous variables that a patient encounters. Gradual changes are a very common cause of chronic disease. Factors that often cause gradual changes include a long list, such as insufficient sleep, lack of water, poor diet or dietary habits, unhealthy lifestyle, too much noise, negative thoughts, unsupportive relationships, pollution and environmental toxins.
- *Progressive* changes are the result of the deterioration of the body over time due to continual stressors and unresolved symptoms or diseases.

Progression of disease occurs when a patient's innate healing ability is blocked or when the signs and symptoms are not adequately addressed for an extended period of time. Death is inevitable, but progressive debility is not. Understanding the progressive nature of disease involves recognizing the interrelationship and reliance of every aspect of the body on every other aspect. The organ systems 'feed' and nurture each other. If one system, or aspect of the body is in a continual state of overwhelm, it will result in a cascade effect on other organ systems. The greater the progression of disease, often the more difficult it is for a patient to return to a state of health. There are times when disease states manifest months or years after physical or emotional trauma to the body. In situations like this there will always be some signs of change in health status, such as changes in the key indicators to health that coincided with the timing of the trauma. When the impact of a situation or trauma has healed, the signs of disharmony will resolve; if, on the other hand, the signs are ignored or the impact of the trauma is suppressed, it is typical for the mild signs and symptoms to progress to a chronic disease state. The rate of progression depends on the accumulation of other health factors, and the intensity of the trauma that is suppressed. An understanding of the interrelationship of anatomy, physiology and pathology, how the body prioritizes functions, and the significance of the different symptom patterns is required to fully understand the progressive changes that occur in the human body.

Case 6.1

A young man finds out that his father was killed in a car accident due to a drunk driver. Shortly after this he starts having digestive problems – bloody stools, chronic diarrhea, lower right quadrant pain, weight loss, gas, increasing fatigue and disrupted sleep. He had no history of digestive problems. There is increasing demand for him to support his family and to take on increased responsibilities and financial burdens. One year later the case is thrown out of court. He finds the situation too upsetting and doesn't talk about it – which indicates a suppressed emotion with a negative charge. As he 'goes on with his life' his digestive concerns continue to get worse. Two years later he is diagnosed with Crohn's disease and within a year ends up having surgery to remove his colon. His digestive symptoms improve initially but his fatigue and insomnia continue to get worse – which indicates a progression of the initial pattern. He also now has the symptoms of being cold more frequently – which indicates a Yin deficiency state and a lack of internal earth. The root cause still needs to be addressed, which means addressing the emotional impact of loss. The greatest and deepest impact will remain in the area of the initial insult, yet the overall effect is wide spread. In order for the body to start to heal, the root cause needs to be addressed as it is 'feeding' the rest.

Intensity

The intensity of symptoms indicates the *degree* of overwhelm or aggravation that accompanies a specific sign or symptom. The intensity is a reflection of the disrupting factor and the susceptibility and strength of the patient at the time of the disruption. The intensity can sometimes be measured quantitatively, such as 'three tablespoons of sputum', however for most systems an analogue scale from 0 to 10 is used, where 0 is the absence of a symptom, 1 is very mild, up to 10 which is extreme. The intensity of symptoms ranges from mild, to moderate, to intense. The greater the intensity, the more important it is to pay attention and to determine what needs to be changed.

- *Mild* symptoms, especially if infrequent, are indications that the body is in a slight overwhelm state. They often are reported as being from 1 to 4 out of 10 on the analog scale. Mild symptoms often are due to deficiencies, excesses, or exposures in a patient's life that have caused a minor disruption in the patient's attempt to adapt and compensate to the factors that it encounters; for example, experiencing bloating after eating a large meal, a headache after too much alcohol, or low back pain when wearing high-heeled shoes. Usually mild symptoms are easily resolved with changes in lifestyle and by addressing aggravating and ameliorating factors.
- *Moderate* symptoms often are reported as being 4 to 7 out of 10 and are the result of mild symptoms that go unaddressed for an extended period of time or due to exposure that is more intense or constant. Moderate symptoms demand more attention and change as they indicate that the internal mechanisms of the body are repeatedly being stressed. If the onset of the symptoms is moderate to start with, there was likely a specific situation, behavior, or event that was disruptive. If moderate symptoms resolve quickly, and on their own, they can indicate an acute healing response or removal of the disrupting factor. For example, a patient might have an intense headache that came on suddenly. If the headache was due to the presence of heavy chemicals, then the headache often will resolve on its own when a patient removes themselves from that situation.
- *Intense* symptoms are reported to be 8 to 10 on the analogue scale. These symptoms often require more immediate attention, especially when they involve vital functions, such as breathing, bleeding, fracture, punctures, abdominal guarding, lack of movement, etc. If the intensity of symptoms came on suddenly it indicates that action needs to be taken immediately. The intensity of symptoms does not always equate to severity or degree of health risk. For example, arthritic pain can be very intense, and very disruptive to a patient's quality of life, but it does not mean that a patient's health is in danger. Symptoms will be intense when the impact of a single situation or incident is high or when there has been exposure to many factors with the same energetic quality all within a short period of time.

Frequency

Symptoms can either be constant, intermittent, or infrequent; this frequency of symptoms indicates the exposure to a factor and the interrelationship and cumulative impact of different factors.

- *Constant* symptoms are either due to a factor that a patient is exposed to daily or indicates a progression of the disease state. For example, if a patient has gas and bloating on a daily basis it is not going to be caused by a food that they eat once a week, it is going to be caused by a food that they eat on a daily basis or it is due to a deeper imbalance in the intestinal flora. The specific type of symptom provides insight into what consistency means, both from the point of view of exposure and of risk to health. For example, chronic back pain can indicate a deeper pathology such as spinal stenosis or metastases of cancer, a recurring imbalanced posture, improper execution of an exercise program, depression, gynecological problems, or muscle strain that has never been addressed (Seller 2000). Symptoms are a road map. If chronic back pain was a chief complaint, then during the intake a practitioner would listen for and ask questions to assist in 'mentally walking backwards' to determine the root cause of the back ache. For example, if it was determined that gynecological problems were contributing to the back ache the next step is to determine what caused the gynecological problems. The process continues until the factors that are being discussed are at the level of the personal essence, the building blocks to health, or at the level of external and environmental factors.
- *Intermittent* symptoms indicate occasional exposure either to a building block to health, such as food, or to environmental, or external factors. They refer to those symptoms that happen a couple times a week or monthly, for example, pain or discomfort after a specific exercise or movement, the onset of gas after eating a specific food, the return of sinusitis when exposed to mold, the onset of a headache when around smoke or strong odors, or monthly cramps associated with menstruation. Intermittent symptoms are influenced by a patient's constitution and susceptibility and indicate the interrelation of different aspects of the body and the cumulative effect of different symptoms. For example, when a patient is tired or hungry, they get a headache or they are short-tempered; or when frustrated they tend to have pain in the area of the gallbladder, which is further aggravated when they eat fatty food or a heavier meal.
- *Infrequent* symptoms relate to those factors that occur rarely. If the severity of the symptoms is mild and the duration is short, the infrequent symptoms often indicate an acute healing response or a period of time when the disrupting factors caused a state of overwhelm. For example, a patient that had poison ivy only once and it resolved within a week without any complications, or a patient who reports that they had insomnia for a month during a period of intense stress. If the infrequent symptom is followed by the onset of other symptoms, or a change in health status, then the cause of the infrequent symptom needs to be identified and addressed, as well as a review of the type of treatments that were used. This type of situation often indicates an incomplete acute healing response or the suppression of a symptom that has resulted in a worsening of the disease state. For example, a patient who contracts a parasite while on vacation and undergoes treatment only for the diarrhea symptoms and then, a year later, reports that his bowels 'have never been right' since his trip. A patient who is physically abused and treats her physical wounds, but ignores the psychological impact and then finds that

she is more short-tempered overall and that her energy is slowly getting worse over time. A patient who injured their shoulder playing sports 3 years ago and still requires anti-inflammatories to manage the pain. Some infrequent events and situations have a profound impact on a patient and require time and processing in order for them to re-establish a sense of health and well being. The more that this process is supported versus rushed or suppressed, the greater the recovery for the patient.

CAUSAL FACTORS

Patients usually seek medical assistance due to the onset or progression of signs and symptoms; the practitioner's role is then to work backwards in order to determine the cause. During an intake, patients reveal two things, the first being their story, the second being the manifestation and nature of their symptoms. A practitioner's role is to correlate the two, and to understand what information is missing or misleading.

Good clinical skills convert subjective symptoms into objective signs. A physical examination yields more signs. Signs are not simply the product of observation; they also contain knowledge (Duffin 2007).

As a practitioner listens to a patient's story, they are initially determining what caused the disruption to health. The next step is to determine the specific factors that play a role. For example a practitioner might surmise that a patient is intolerant to certain foods as they have infrequent, mild gas and bloating, but based on the symptoms alone a practitioner does not know the specific food or foods that are the cause or why the digestive system is an area of susceptibility. It is only by listening and questioning the patient that this information can be revealed.

There is sometimes one cause or initiating factor, but often, especially in chronic disease, there are multiple factors that have contributed or aggravated the situation. For example, a patient may have lung cancer and their 30-year history of heavy smoking may be deemed the primary cause, but their outlook on life and their lifestyle might also be factors. What the practitioner is listening for, and looking for, are the patterns that correlate and resonate together. Signs and symptoms 'carry' the same pattern as the disrupting factors. Each factor has specific qualities and attributes and the symptoms that manifest carry these same characteristics. The location and nature of the symptoms depends on the particular disrupting factors and the part of the patient that mirrors that cause.

In many textbooks on differential diagnoses, the cause of a symptom is listed as other physical symptoms or pathological states. For example, 'The common causes of abdominal pain include gastroenteritis, gastritis, peptic ulcer disease, reflux esophagitis, irritable bowel syndrome, dysmenorrhea…' (Seller 2000). This information is valuable, but from a naturopathic perspective it does not equate to the cause of disease. The causes of symptoms and disease occur on the level of the personal essence, the building blocks to health, and the external and environmental level. The cause of disease is not another symptom or pathology.

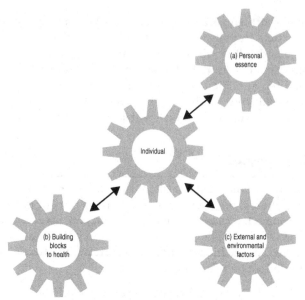

Fig 6.1 Causal factors. The individual manifests the disruption, but the cause does not originate on this level. The initial causes of signs and symptoms originate from (a) the personal essence, (b) the building blocks to health, and (c) external and environmental factors.

The disruption of health arises due to three main factors (see Fig. 6.1):

1. Disharmony between a patient's life and their personal essence.
2. The continual disharmony in the building blocks to health or constant exposure to disrupting external or environmental factors. This results in subtle symptoms that progressively increase until there is a disruption on the psychological plane, a deterioration of bodily function, or a weakening of structures.
3. A situation, event, or external threat of such intensity that it overwhelms the body quickly.

The progression of disease itself, can also be a factor when the initial signs and symptoms are not being adequately addressed, or due to a weakened vitality and healing potential of a patient.

Disharmony with the personal essence

The personal essence is a patient's foundation, their blueprint; it represents their core. The stronger a patient's core, the more their life is in tune with their core, the greater the sense of health and stronger the healing potential of the body. A patient's beliefs and expectations for themselves and for their life are reflected in their personal essence. When there is a lack of harmony or achievement based on these expectations, a patient often will feel a sense of discontentment or will have a gnawing feeling that just doesn't go away.

A patient might have periods of being 'okay', but a pattern or sense of un-fulfillment will continue to creep into their consciousness. There often is an unrelenting sense of being unsettled or dissatisfied and there tends to be chaos and disruption in getting things accomplished; for example, a patient finds that their work is no longer satisfying, the opportunity to move up in the company seems further away and the promise of new responsibilities doesn't materialize. Situations that they were okay with in the past now bother them and they don't have the same sense of fulfillment. Ultimately it indicates that their 'measuring stick', that is their core, is not in line with their life. Sometimes disharmony at this level is addressed by changing expectations and beliefs, other times it involves making life changes, sometimes drastic ones.

Most people, in retrospect, recognize that the sequence of events in their life are filled with synchronicity and have resulted in opportunities that they didn't realize at the time. For example, they met their spouse at their new job after they were let go unexpectedly; or the time they missed their plane, they were needed at home. We often think of symptoms arising as a result of something that is happening or that has happened. Disharmony at the level of personal essence can result because of something that is going to happen. The personal essence is the internal guide, it is what connects people on a spiritual plane or on the level of the collected consciousness, and it has the ability to make decisions without the parameter of time. Life is like a play, and the personal essence is aware that in the upcoming act your role is changing, and hence you need to make changes in the present, in order to be ready for your new role in the future.

Some holistic forms of medicine, such as homeopathy, believe that most chronic diseases originate at the level of the personal essence (Vithoulkas 1981). There is a belief that situations 'happen for a reason' in order to keep us on our journey and our path. The personal essence permeates all aspects of a patient, but often we think of it being most closely linked to the unconscious psychological aspect and linked to the greater collective consciousness.

Case 6.2

A 37-year-old female is married with two children. She loves her life and her family, has a successful job and is active in her community. She is considered fun loving, happy, and content by friends and family. Yet, she has a constant internal feeling of not being confident or good enough. She is surprised, even embarrassed when she gets promoted at work and she never informs any of her friends of her promotion. She is cautious with reprimanding her children, as she fears she will be perceived as a bad parent. During the intake she talks about growing up in a house where everything had to be perfect, and getting top grades and being the best in any sport she participated in was expected. As an adult she recognizes that she doesn't agree with the 'rules' that she grew up with. A treatment focused on reframing her sense of what is meant to be confident allowed her to feel better about herself and increased her enjoyment in life. This was accomplished through awareness exercises, journaling, and self-evaluation exercises of current situations.

The building blocks to health

The building blocks represent those lifestyle factors – nutrition, water, sleep, exercise – and behaviors – breathing, posture, fresh air, mental attitude – that provide a patient with the nutrients and qualities that they require to sustain life (refer to Chapter 3). Many diseases, especially chronic diseases, are due to the wear-and-tear of having to cope with the constant lifestyle excesses and deficiencies that eventually cause the body to 'break down'. For example, a history of eating poorly, not drinking sufficient water, being too sedentary, of poor posture, ineffective breathing, not enough fresh air or sleep and relaxation, or holding onto thoughts and emotions that are unhealthy.

> We are medicating the effect of living disharmoniously. We are trying to treat the effects of disharmony rather than treating the cause of disharmony (Mitchell 2007).

A healthy lifestyle also involves living a life that is in tune with the rhythms of nature. There is a rhythm to sunrise and sunset, the lunar cycle, birth and death. This rhythm is mirrored in the ebb and flow of the body and provides a guide for behavior and lifestyle. For example, melatonin is the principal hormone responsible for synchronization of sleep and it follows a circadian cycle (Smale et al 2008). Many metabolic processes, including blood pressure and respiration, also follow a circadian rhythm (Alagiakrishnan et al 2001, Tu 2006). When a patient is living a lifestyle that is more in tune with the natural rhythms, health is more easily maintained and achieved. The physiological demands of the body change throughout life and adjusting eating habits, exercise and lifestyle to correspond with age is an important aspect of staying in rhythm with life.

The building blocks to health include acknowledging and honoring the natural urges of the body; such as urination, hunger, burping, thirst, strong breathing or panting due to exercise, passing gases, bowel movements, ejaculation of semen, yawning, vomiting, sneezing, tears, and sleep (Lad 1998). These natural urges are an internal mechanism of the body to adjust to states of excess, deficiency, or disharmony. The suppression of these urges inhibits the body's natural ability to bring about balance and contributes to symptom and disease processes.

Addressing these building blocks is part of every treatment plan. In many situations, especially when the healing potential of a patient is high, the most efficient way to restore a homeodynamic state might be to simply address the building blocks. Even when the building blocks are just an aggravating factor and not the initiating factor, addressing them often will increase the patient's overall sense of wellness, decrease the progression of disease, and increase the motivation and drive to make any other necessary changes.

External and environmental factors

Life events

Sometimes there is a direct correlation between a situation and the onset of symptoms, for example in times of crisis, when there is an accident or when we hear bad news. When a patient reports that their health has been worse ever since a specific date or period of time then it is likely that a specific event was the catalyst or it was due to a patient's response to an event. The impact of a specific situation depends on a patient's current state of health at the time that the situation occurs, the severity of the situation and the constitution and previous life experiences of a patient.

Man does not simply perceive things, but also perceives the meaning of things. Meaning precedes perception. That which does not mean anything is not, as a rule, perceived. Perception and retention are vital adaptive functions. They are not aimed at meaningless events (Thass-Theinemann 1968).

When a situation or life event overwhelms a patient, time seems to slow down, as if the state of overwhelm suspends everything.

Beyond the rarefied atmosphere of academic biomedicine, most people can recall special moments that tell them that there is more to life than usually meets the eye. During emergency or life-threatening situations, for example, 'time seems to slow down' to allow quicker responses than usual (Oshman 2003).

The degree of impact is mirrored in the degree of shift away from health. How a patient handles a life event determines the ongoing impact that it will have on their healing potential and susceptibility to becoming overwhelmed in the future. For example, it is natural to initially go through a stage of distress, such as pain after being in an accident, or the sense of grief when someone close to you dies. However, if a patient becomes stuck in the situation – either due to not addressing the initiating factor, or choosing treatments that palliate and suppress versus cure – and the symptoms do not resolve, then it creates or intensifies an area of susceptibility and increases the likelihood of recurring symptoms. For example, when a patient becomes 'trapped' in grief, they are likely to be triggered to a greater degree when other situations of grief arise. If the patient remains angry because of an accident that was caused by a careless driver, they are more likely to be overly cautious or nervous when they drive, and they are more likely to become angry in other situations that display a similar pattern, for example a situation where someone is careless and steps in front of them because they are distracted by talking on their cell phone.

It is not the situation itself that impacts health, it is the patient's response to that situation. A patient's mind has the capacity to change reality, to expand the truth or to forget – hence it dictates the obstacle and the challenge that must be dealt with. For example, a patient is driving home from a trip with her son in the backseat – all of a sudden a truck coming towards her swerves out of its lane and into hers – she brakes suddenly – pulls off to the shoulder – the car behind her brakes suddenly and swerves – she think she is going to be hit, the truck driver recognizes his error and pulls back into his own lane – just missing her car. No accident happened. No one hit someone else. The impact depends on how her mind stores the story – did she almost die, or did she react quickly and everything was fine. If she interprets the situation as she 'almost died', the psychological state overrides the reality of the situation and results in functional and structural changes. This is very common in post-traumatic stress disorders. You know when a situation still 'triggers' a patient as their emotional state changes when they discuss the situation, or they actively avoid discussing the situation.

Social aspects

The *social* aspect of life is where people spend most of their time. It relates to one's family, community, and work. The dynamics and demands of each can contribute to one's health or to one's disease. It is helpful to recognize how each one affects a patient, and what their motivation and expectations are of each. Understanding the impact of the social aspect of a patient's life involves seeing the role that they play in their different social environments and realizing that when they are 'triggered' by situations or people often it indicates something that they have to address, not something that needs to change in someone else. The balance between family, community, and work often is an area of struggle or discontentment for people. That struggle, if not resolved, can contribute to increased symptoms and ultimately to disease.

External factors

Many of today's diseases and health problems are linked to an over-burden of toxins in the body. Toxins and harmful chemicals are everywhere: car exhaust fumes, factory smoke, cigarette smoke, the chemical in patient care products, hair dyes, household and kitchen products, cleaning products, products for our lawns and homes, and products and chemicals used in manufacturing and industry. The body is constantly being bombarded with 'foreign' and toxic chemicals and substances that enter the body through the air we breathe, the water we drink, the food we eat and what we put on our skin. In normal internal functioning, the body will 'take-in' substances, keep what it needs and excrete the rest. The body is unfamiliar with many of these chemicals and unable to naturally excrete them. Foreign chemicals often result in modifications of body functions, such as the hormone disrupting impact of plastics (phenols), or they accumulate in tissues and organs disrupting the normal functioning of these body signals (Bonefeld-Jørgensen 2007, Calafat et al 2008, Krüger et al 2008).

> It is also known that many toxins undergo bioaccumulation through the food chain and that synergistic effects can occur whereby combinations of toxins can be more potent than the sum of patient toxins (Cohen 2007).

Nutritional status impacts susceptibility to chemical exposure and the presence of toxic chemicals is intensified by chronic dehydration and diets and lifestyles that are not conducive to aiding excretion, resulting in negative changes to health (Kordas et al 2007).

Other environmental influences that are impacting health are the abuse and over-use of computers, television, cell-phones, and other electromagnetic fields (EMF)-producing devices. Spending hours in front of a computer or television often is correlated with being more sedentary, obesity, vision problems, and neck and low back pain (Bhanderi et al 2006, Bali et al 2007, Alricsson et al 2008, Rey-López et al 2008). The use of computer games has been associated with hyperactivity disorders (Dworak et al 2007). Cell phones and EMF devices are correlated with headaches, brain cancer and other health concerns (Williams 2005, Djeridance et al 2008, Hardell & Sage 2008).

Medical interventions

Medical interventions, of all types, are a required and valuable aspect of medicine. Yet, some interventions and the use of drugs to suppress symptoms contribute to, and cause, disease. Adverse-effects of medications are often treated with additional drugs, which in turn can cause additional problems. When the symptoms are suppressed, versus the root causes addressed, the disease is forced deeper into the body. The deeper within the body the disease is, the greater the impact on health. A skin rash for example often is a sign that an organ system of the body is over loaded. The rash is a way of the body excreting the toxins without harming the organ. When drugs or treatments are used that suppress the rash, the toxins are forced back into the body and often result in deeper pathologies (Greaves 2005). Another example is anxiety. The anxiety is an indication that there needs to be a change on some level, that for some reason the body is unsettled. It might be because of the food a patient is eating, a job they need to leave, or a new opportunity that they need to go after. If medication to decrease the uneasiness is prescribed, without awareness of what is behind it, the message is the suppressed and the change that needs to be made isn't made. The uneasiness goes deeper affecting the body at a deeper level and when you stop the medication the uneasiness often is still there.

Medical interventions play a valuable role in saving lives and addressing high risk health situations. The concern with these interventions, however, is when they are employed instead of, or in place of, addressing the underlying initiating and aggravating factors of disease, especially when the risk to health is low or moderate.

REFERENCES

Alagiakrishnan K, Masaki K, Schatz I, Curb JD, Blanchette PL 2001 Blood pressure dysregulation syndrome. The case for control throughout the circadian cycle. Geriatrics 56(3):50–52, 55–56, 59–60

Alricsson M, Landstad BJ, Romild U, Gundersen KT 2008 Physical activity, health, BMI and body complaints in high school students. Minerva Pediatr 60(1):19–25

Bali J, Navin N, Thakur BR 2007 Computer vision syndrome: A study of the knowledge, attitudes and practices in Indian Ophthalmologists. Indian J Ophthalmol 55:289–294

Benor DJ 2006 Wholistic Healing, The Healing Potential in a Word – part III. Positive Health, Portsmouth

Bhanderi DJ, Choudhary S, Doshi VG 2006 A community-based study of asthenopia in computer operators. Indian J Ophthalmol 56:51–55

Bonefeld-Jørgensen EC, Long M, Hofmeister MV, Vinggaard AM 2007 Endocrine-disrupting potential of bisphenol A, bisphenol A dimethacrylate, 4-*n*-nonylphenol, and 4-*n*-octylphenol in vitro: new data and a brief review. Environm Health Perspect, 115(l):69–76

Bridges L 2004 Face Reading in Chinese Medicine. Churchill Livingstone, Missouri

Calafat AM, Ye X, Wong LY, Reidy JA, Needham LL 2008 Exposure of the U.S. Population to Bisphenol A and 4-tertiary-Octylphenol:2003–2004. Environment Health Perspect 116(1):39–44

Cohen M 2007 'Detox': science or sales pitch? Aust Fam Physician 36(12):1009–1010

Collins RD 1997 Differential Diagnosis in Primary Care, second edition. Lippincott, Philadelphia

Djeridance Y, Touitou Y, de Seze R 2008 Influence of electromagnetic fields emitted by GSM-900 cellular telephones on the circadian patterns of gonadal, adrenal and pituitary hormones in men. Radiat Res 169(3):337–343

Duffin J 2007 History of Medicine. University of Toronto Press, Toronto

Dworak M, Schierl T, Bruns T, Strüder HK 2007 Impact of singular excessive computer game and television exposure on sleep patterns and memory performance of school-aged children. Pediatrics 120(5):978–985

Greaves MW 2005 Antihistamines in dermatology. Skin Pharmacol Physiol 18(5):220–229

Hardell L, Sage C 2008 Biological effects from electromagnetic field exposure and public exposure standards. Biomed Pharmacother 62(2):104–109

Kordas K, Lönnerdal B, Stoltzfus RJ 2007 Interactions between nutrition and environmental exposures: effects on health outcomes in women and children. J Nutr 137(12):2794–2797

Krüger T, Long M Bonefeld-Jørgensen EC 2008 Plastic components affect the activation of the aryl hydrocarbon and the androgen receptor. Toxicology 246 (2–3):112–123

Lad V 1998 Ayurveda, the Science of Self-healing. Motilal Banarsidass Publishers, Delhi

Lad V 2005 Ayurvedic Perspectives on Selected Pathologies. The Ayurvedic Press, New Mexico

Mitchell B 2007 The Vis Part 1 and 2. Presented at the First International Editors Retreat, Foundations of Naturopathic Medicine Project

Morgan WL, Engel GL 1969 The Clinical Approach to the Patient. WB Saunders, Philadelphia

Oschman J 2003 Energy Medicine in Therapeutics and Human Performance. Butterworth-Heinemann, Edinburgh

Rey-López JP, Vincente-Rodríguez G, Biosca M, Moreno LA 2008 Sedentary behaviour and obesity development in children and adolescents. Nutr Metab Cardiovasc Dis 18(3):242–251

Seller RH 2000 Differential Diagnosis of Common Complaints, fourth edition. WB Saunders Company, Philadelphia

Smale L, Nunez AA, Schwartz MD 2008 Rhythms in a diurnal brain. Biol Rhythm Res 39(3):305–318

Thass-Theinemann T 1968 Symbolic Behavior. Washington Square Press, New York

Tu BP, McKnight SL 2006 Metabolic cycles as an underlying basis of biological oscillations. www.nature.com/reviews/molcellbio Vol 7

Vithoulkas G 1981 The Science of Homeopathy. Grove Press, New York

Williams RM 2005 Cell Phones and Children. Townsend Letter July 26–28

FURTHER READING

Bartra J, Mullol J, del Cuvillo, et al 2007 Air pollution and allergens. J Invest Allergol Clin Immunol 17(2):3–8

Beers MH, Berkow R 1999 The Merck Manual of Diagnosis and Therapy. Merck Research Laboratories, New Jersey

Capra F 1982 The Turning Point, Science, Society, and the Rising Culture. Bantam Books, Toronto

Davenport S, Goldberg D, Miller T 1987 How psychiatric disorders are missed during medical consultations. Lancet 2:439–441

Goldfield GS, Mallory R, Parker T 2007 Effects of modifying physical activity and sedentary behaviour on psychosocial adjustment in overweight/obese children. J Pediatr Psychol 2007 32(7):783–793

Houston MC 2007 The role of mercury and cadmium heavy metals in vascular disease, hypertension, coronary heart disease, and myocardial infarction. Alt Ther Health Med 13(2):128–133

Lindlahr H 1975 Philosophy of Natural Therapeutics. CW Daniel Company, UK

Lloyd IR 2006 Messages From the Body, a Guide to the Energetics of Health. Naturopathic Publications, Toronto

Lynes MA, Kang TJ, Sensi ST, Perdrizet GA, Hightower LE 2007 Heavy metal ions in normal physiology, toxic stress, and cytoprotection. Ann N Y Acad Sci 1113:159–172

Rogers C 1961 On Becoming a Patient. Mifflin, Boston

Straker LM, O'Sullivan PB, Smith A, Perry M 2007 Computer use and habitual spinal posture in Australian adolescents. Public Health Reports 122(5):632–643

CHAPTER 7
Health and disease

How practitioners define health and disease, and their expectations and beliefs about wellness, influences every aspect of assessment, diagnosis, and treatment. It dictates what information is sought and how it is interpreted. It determines whether the emphasis of the patient–practitioner relationship is on addressing the factors that caused the disease or just treating the symptoms. Whether health and disease are viewed as logical or random, and whether a practitioner is trained to integrate all aspects of a patient or just address specific pathological conditions, impacts the meaning that is assigned to symptoms and diseases and the approach used.

Health and disease are not two separate states of being. They are a continuum. This continuum allows a patient to move from a state of health to disease or from disease to health. At any point in time, if vitality, willingness, and the building blocks to health are present, a patient's innate healing power works to sustain life and restore health. The naturopathic definition of health and disease is based on the concepts of holism and vitalism. It recognizes the uniqueness of patients and the logic of health and disease. In naturopathic medicine, the practitioner's role is to guide patients back to health, with the recognition that true healing is an inherent ability and right within everyone.

No doctor since the beginning of time has ever cured a patient. No doctor ever will, for Nature alone can cure. Physicians are not meant to work wonders or perform miracles. A true physician is a teacher who helps his or her patients work through their problems at all levels. Doctors are meant to use their knowledge of the patient's past illnesses and present conditions to intuit future possibilities for health and establish a healing strategy for the patient. True physicians leave the miracles to Nature, offering themselves as channels through which Nature can work her magic (Svoboda 1989).

HEALTH – THE HOMEODYNAMIC STATE

The natural, or desirable, state of existence, is health. In a healthy state, the waves of a patient are in sync. Health is order; disease is disorder. 'It is determined by the quantity, quality, and distribution of the body's constituents and the harmonious interaction of the organ networks' (Beinfield & Korngold 1991). A patient's view of health and disease changes as they mature and age, as a result of life experiences and the perception of what is healthy or not is also affected culture, religion, economics, race, class, gender, and other social and biological factors (Duffin 2007).

Health is an attitude, and the desirability of the outcome depends on one's beliefs, expectations, and upbringing. For some this means the absence of signs or symptoms in the functional and structural aspects of the body; for others it represents an awakening on a psychological or spiritual level. For others health is the absence of any symptoms that impact daily life; with the tolerance for symptoms varying greatly. Some people perceive themself as healthy, even when they are aware that they have a disease or disability (Justice 1998). In this book, health is defined as the harmonious vibration of the psychological, functional, and structural aspects of a patient with their personal essence and their external environment.

The study of human health must include a wider perspective than just a patient. Human beings are not isolated entities; they are born, live, and die, inseparable from the larger contexts of physical, social, political, and spiritual influences (Vithoulkas 1981). The study of human health needs to include, at a minimum, a patient's lifestyle, their habits, the environment in which they life, their work, their community, and a patient's sense of spirituality or inner life force. A patient's assessment of their own health is a better predictor of their mortality than a physician's evaluations or laboratory tests (Idler & Kasl 1991). Hence, understanding what a patient views as health, and where they see themselves on the continuum of health and disease is an essential part of the assessment process.

To understand how a patient shifts from a state of health to one of disease it is helpful to first understand how they maintain health. Human beings are complex, non-linear, self-organizing systems that constantly exchange energy with their surroundings in a dynamic process in order to maintain themselves (Rubik 2005 in Louise 2007). They are continuously responding to, compensating for, and balancing the various internal and external stimuli that they encounter. There are periods of development, growth, and maturation as they are continually replacing, healing, and nourishing every aspect of themselves. There is continual change and movement in both the tangible and intangible aspects of human life. Throughout all of this, the aim is to maintain a homeodynamic state.

Human beings go through cycles in their lives similar to the seasons in nature – beginning in birth and ending in death, with stages of growth, maturity, and decay in between (Beinfield & Korngold 1991).

Factors that assist in maintaining health include living a life in alignment with one's constitution, paying attention to the 'little' signs and symptoms, and addressing them as they arise.

The question of health or disease often comes down to patient responsibility. In this context, responsibility means choosing a healthy alternative over a less healthy one. If you want to be healthy, simply make healthy choices (Murray & Pizzorno 1991).

The responsibility of each patient is to provide the building blocks to health; the body knows how to do the rest. The primary goal of naturopathic medicine is to enhance the innate healing potential of a patient, and restore the normal harmonic state of health by addressing the factors of disease and tuning the body as a unit. Health is more than just the absence of disease; it is a vital dynamic state which enables a patient to adapt to, and thrive in a wide range of environments and stresses. For example, people who 'catch' every cold that comes by are not healthy when they are symptom free; they can be considered healthy only when they stop being overly susceptible to infection (Murray & Pizzorno 1991).

Key indicators of health

Every component of a patient functions autonomously to some degree, yet it is interdependent on every other component in the body. For example, the digestive system has its own internal control mechanism, yet it is impacted by the nervous system, the respiratory system, and every other system of the body. If one component of the patient is in a state of deficiency or excess, it will impact other components. As a result, other aspects compensate to ensure that vital organs and functions are preserved. Through feedback loops, internal cellular processes, and the constant exchange of energy, a patient is able to handle tremendous fluctuation before becoming overwhelmed.

When imbalances in lifestyle or environment exceed a patient's ability to compensate or adapt appropriately, it causes a state of overwhelm or exhaustion; and hence there is a shift away from health. These shifts are initially subtle. What shifts and how it shifts relate to a patient's constitution, the disruptive factors, and how a patient attempted to compensate. Likewise, as the lifestyle and environmental factors improve, there is a return back toward health. The shift, away from or towards health, initially appears in one of six physiological functions. These functions are indicators or 'warning signs' that something is out of balance. They represent common symptoms that are linked to many organ systems and bodily functions. These key indicators to health include: the elimination of waste products, sleep, appetite and thirst, temperature regulation, mood, and overall energy level. When assessing the key indicators with a patient it is important to understand what is typically 'normal' for a patient, and what has changed. The 'normal' state depends on a patient's constitution, age, and the progression of disease.

Elimination of wastes

A patient has many ways of eliminating the waste products that are produced by the body. Urine, stools, carbon dioxide, and sweat are the primary waste products produced. In order to maintain optimal function, a patient must be able to eliminate their wastes on an ongoing basis (Frawley 1989). In most Eastern medical systems, and in naturopathic medicine, one of the first steps in treatment is to ensure that the routes of elimination are open and functioning appropriately and adequately.

The waste products of the body serve physiological functions and are essential to their respective organs. The urinary system removes the water, salt, nitrogenous wastes, and other substances and is required to maintain the normal concentration of electrolytes within the bodily fluids. For example, excessive urination decreases perspiration production and excessive perspiring results in a scanty volume of urine. Excessive perspiration reduces body temperature and creates dehydration. In the same way, too much urination creates dehydration and causes coldness of the hands and feet (Lad 1998).

Sleep

Sleep can be disrupted by many factors, such as: poor dietary habits, ingestion of stimulants, like caffeine and sugar; excessive mental activity, too much physical activity right before bedtime, musculoskeletal pain, poor sleep environment, stress, excessive television or computer usage, too much noise or light, shift work, a sense of discontentment at one's core, or it can be affected by deeper pathologies, such as anaemia. Sleep is required for healing and repair. In a healthy state, sleep follows the circadian rhythm which is linked to the natural day–night cycle (Roehrs & Roth 2008). What is normal, with respect to sleep, for each patient depends on their constitution. What is noteworthy is when the normal pattern of sleep changes or when the sleep pattern is not conducive to health.

Appetite and thirst

A noticeable increase or decrease in a patient's typical appetite or thirst, or a patient's pattern of eating, is a sign that needs to be explored further. Water, food, and air are the primary nutrients required to sustain life and 'feed' the body. Thirst and appetite depend on a patient's digestive fire, previous water and food intake, and physical activity level. Cravings, excess desire for food or water, or lack of desire often are indicators of deeper issues. Based on a patient's constitution each patient has also 'normal' level of appetite and thirst. The type and amount of food and water depends on a patient's current level of health, the current season, and the level of activity that they are involved in (Maciocia 1989).

Temperature regulation

A patient's constitution dictates their normal body temperature. Temperature normally shifts in response to internal and external conditions and with health and disease. For example, sweating is a natural response that is designed to decrease core body temperature in response to an increase in external temperature; shivering does the opposite. It is important to be able to regulate body temperature according to internal and external changes. When body temperature is not 'normal', such as constantly being cold in the core, cold or warm hands and feet, profuse sweating, or isolated cold parts of the body, it often is an indication of a deeper problem.

Mood

For many patients the first sign that they are 'off' is that their mood shifts. There is an altered feeling that something isn't right. Each patient has a tendency to certain moods; for example, for some people if they are having an 'off' day they are likely to be irritable, others sad, and others more anxious.

Energy level

A patient's sense of energy is a subjective quality. What one patient views as having a high amount of energy another patient might view as low. What is important is when the amount of 'normal' energy for a patient changes. How and when the energy changes provides information as to the factors that have affected energy. For example, some patients experience low energy after a large meal, for others it drops after specific foods, and for some energy increases after eating. Having great energy when you wake up that decreases throughout the day tells a practitioner a different story than if a patient wakes up with low energy that stays low all day long. For some energy level is dependent on what a patient is doing or who they are with. The impact of exercise on energy also is valuable in understanding what the message of low energy is conveying.

Healing potential

A patient's healing potential is a reflection of their patient essence. It is determined by their constitution, life experiences, and their will to live.

Constitution + Life experiences = Susceptibility

Susceptibility + Will power = Healing potential

A patient has an overall healing potential, as does each part and component of the body. For example, it is possible that the healing potential or vitality of a patient is strong, yet the vitality of a specific organ is weak such as a vibrant and healthy kidney in a man who just died of a heart attack:

The kidney has no value to the man, and in spite of its own inherent vitality, very rapidly loses significance. By the same token, a dysfunctional kidney can affect the vitality of a man with an otherwise extremely vital heart; if both kidneys fail, the vitality of the system fails (Mitchell 2007).

Healing potential is impacted by a patient's age, their beliefs and expectations, and by the severity and type of disease itself. Some patients are born with a strong constitution; they have the ability to fight disease and withstand a lot of stress without it significantly affecting their overall wellness. Other patients are more sensitive and have a greater degree of inner weakness and susceptibility. The impact of specific incidences, the accumulation of life experiences, and lifestyle factors all have the potential to create areas of susceptibility. For example, if a patient injures their knee playing sports and the injury doesn't heal completely, their knee becomes an area of weakness.

Susceptibility is also affected by a patient's beliefs and thoughts. If a patient believes that disease and a lower level of health come with age, a decrease in healing potential might be more a reflection of this belief than their actual health status. If a patient believes that they are likely to suffer the same symptoms and diseases as their parents, it is more likely to happen. Also, the will to live directly affects healing potential and a loss of will might be much more disastrous to health than any disease.

Constitution

All patients are unique, with different builds, body compositions, and attitudes. Much of western medicine has been based on the principle that because each patient has similar parts, they can be treated the same. Naturopathic medicine, as well as the eastern medicines, recognizes that it is the uniqueness of patients and the integration of all the parts that holds the key to achieving and maintaining health.

A patient's constitution is their baseline, their starting point. It represents their natural tendencies, their primary makeup, their appearance, and their disposition. It represents their inherent strengths and their weaknesses. It can be thought of as the energetic blueprint of their personal essence. A patient's basic constitution is determined at conception, but it is also influenced throughout life due to learned behavior and patient experiences.

From an Ayurvedic medicine perspective, a patient's constitution is inborn and governs all the biological, psychological and physiopathological functions of the body, mind and consciousness. A patient's constitution determines their temperament, natural urges and personal preferences for foods, flavors, temperatures and so on (Lad 1998).

From a Chinese medicine perspective a patient's constitutional strength and resistance comes from their essence. This essence is composed of the prenatal essence and the postnatal essence. The prenatal essence reflects the blending of energies at conception and it determines each patient's basic constitutional make-up, strength, and vitality. It is what makes each patient unique. The postnatal essence is derived from food, drink, and air. It is a reflection of a patient's lifestyle. The overall essence determines growth, reproduction, development, maturation, conception and physiological functions (Maciocia 1989).

Constitution is a way of describing a patient's energetic qualities. Terms such as hot/cold, dry/moist or air/fire/water/earth are used. Patients are complex systems and the qualities that they naturally possess vary on the psychological, functional and structural aspects. For example, a patient can have an *earth* body build – square, solid, thick – an *air* mind – quick, many thoughts, spontaneous – and have high internal *fire* – quick digestion and metabolism, and a tendency to be hot and excitable. The section in the book on Energetic Patterns (Chapter 5) provides a detailed breakdown of these qualities and how they might manifest in different constitutions. Recognizing the constitutional uniqueness of each patient is the basis of disease prevention, health maintenance, and longevity enhancement. It is also an integral part of the treatment of disease.

The energetic qualities used to define a patient's constitution are also used to explain all other aspects of life. The ways in which the qualities of a patient and the qualities in their life interact determine whether the interaction is helpful or harmful. These energetic qualities work on the concept of like increases like and opposites balance each other. If a patient has a 'fire' or 'hot' constitution they are more prone to feel warm, to express feelings of frustration or irritation, to be outgoing and lively, to have symptoms that manifest as red, itchy, hot, or burning. Their digestive system often is an area of susceptibility and they are more likely to be aggravated in hot weather, with hot spicy food, in situations where there is a lot of outward anger or frustration, and when there is intense activity for a long period of time.

A patient's constitutional strength indicates their healing potential and their resistance to disease. For some, their constitution is weak, and they struggle with different diseases throughout their life; while others experience health most of their life. The strength of the constitution is a reflection of the energies derived from the parents and the accumulation of life experiences. Healing potential is strengthened when a patient knows how to live a life that balances, and is in harmony with, their constitution.

A patient's constitution also drives the treatment process. As the baseline, it provides the practitioner with a guide as to how far the patient has swayed away from their starting point. The further away that someone is from their baseline, typically the more disrupted their health. The aim of any treatment is to return to a healthy, homeodynamic constitutional state.

Although you may not like your constitutional proclivities they are yours, and like mooching kinfolk they will stick with you as long as you live. You may as well learn to live with them, and learn how to change your life so you can be as healthy as you possibly can (Svoboda 1989).

Susceptibility

Susceptibility is not separate from constitution, but is a component of it. A patient's susceptibility represents their tendencies, both their strengths and their weaknesses, and is reflected in the healing potential of the body. The aim of maintaining health is supporting and maintaining your areas of strength, and adjusting and balancing for your areas of weakness. For example, a patient who has a strong mind and is academically inclined is best to support this. Some patients find that their health concerns are due to them not recognizing or honoring their strengths.

When a child is young, parents quickly learn whether they are susceptible to specific foods, to certain temperatures, or to certain behaviors. Susceptibilities at this stage might reflect maternal deficiencies, consequences due to the delivery, or might simply be reflective of the child's own constitution. Susceptibilities that indicate preferences, such as right- versus left-handedness, intolerance to a single food, or the desire to be held or not, provide a guide as to what is healthy for that patient, and are best honored. The aim is learn how to live a life that harmonizes and balances the inherent susceptibilities. Susceptibilities in children that indicate a disease state, such as intolerance to a wide number of foods, frequent infections, constant need to be held, or constant crying indicate a disease or heterodynamic state and need to be treated.

Throughout life, even when healthy, a patient displays certain areas of susceptibility; specific aspects that commonly manifest signs of overwhelm or disease. For example, a patient has a tendency to be cold and feels worse when they eat food that is substantially cold or raw; they are also aggravated when it is raining or dull outside. It is common for someone to report that they have problems with their skin whenever they are 'off', or whenever they are stressed their sleep is disrupted. Some people are more likely to have nervous system problems, others digestive or cardiovascular, and so on. Areas of susceptibility provide a guide and indicate the type of lifestyle, diet and emotional factors that a patient needs to pay attention to in order to maintain or achieve health. When susceptibilities have developed over time, the aim of treatment is to restore the inherent strength and resilience to the area, to remove the disrupting factors, to address the root causes, to support or strengthen the underlying organ or system, and to repair any damage that might have occurred.

THE ENERGETICS OF HEALTH

Susceptibilities often are thought of, not in relationship to a patient, but in relationship to specific aspects of a patient such as a susceptible immune system, digestive system, or emotional tendency. Susceptibility refers to the ability of different aspects of a patient to resist disease, to adjust and compensate to disturbing factors, and to heal. A patient's constitution indicates the susceptibilities they are born with. However, susceptibilities also arise over time because of aggravating lifestyle factors, life experiences that eventually take a toll on the body, and isolated situations and incidences that have had a significant impact. Unresolved symptoms or diseases either create an area of weakness or intensify an existing area of susceptibility. An example is a patient who claims that ever since their accident 5 years ago they have a tendency to have weakness or numbness on their left side. Or a patient who catches colds more easily ever since they had a bad chest infection; or a patient who states that their blood pressure has been high ever since their divorce. When there is an increase in susceptibility after a specific event, situation, or acute illness, it is valuable for a practitioner to look at the impact that the situation had and whether it is still impacting the patient. Also, look at how the symptoms manifested and how they were treated. What you are looking for is whether the underlying cause was ever addressed and whether all aspects of a patient were supported and allowed to heal.

DISEASE – THE HETERODYNAMIC STATE

The heterodynamic state is one of disease. It indicates a disruption to the homeodynamic state, that is the waves of the body are out of sync, and the communication flow has broken down (McTaggart 2002). In the ancient Greek model of health, there is one disease. It is called 'dys-ease' or in a real sense, death of ease (Lipton 2005). Some people are able to define a point in time that their health shifted. For others, it is a more gradual progression over a longer period of time. For everyone the balance between health and disease oscillates over a lifetime. The concept of disease, like health, depends on the expectations and beliefs of a patient. For example, some people view disease as the onset of symptoms, and others view themselves as having a disease only when their health concerns disrupt their life or their sense of well being.

Over time, the emphasis of assessment and diagnosis of disease, especially in conventional medicine, has moved from the subjective to the objective. There is great value in objective measurements. They have allowed for the early detection of disease states and have provided a tremendous in-depth understanding of cellular processes. The concern, for many health practitioners, is not the advancement of objective measurements, but the disregard or minimizing of the subjective – the removal of the patient as central and key to diagnosis.

Having worked so hard to objectify illness, do we not have trouble confronting the fullness of the human context in which illness occurs? Have we not, in some consequential way, made disease our focus instead of sick people? (Baron 1985).

In naturopathic medicine, what a patient experiences and how they experience it is key to understanding the significance of any findings and to determining the best treatment strategy. When we desire the ability to 'observe' the inner workings of the body so intently, without an appreciation for how the body innately heals or operates, we run the risk of mistaking a disease state for a healing process. When a patient has no subjective signs of disease, that is, they feel healthy and the key indicators to health are strong or improving, why does an objective measurement 'override' the subjective? As practitioners we need to allow the body room 'to work', while providing ways to support the inherent healing process. There is a fine line between supporting the healing ability of the body and overriding it.

There are times when the structural changes are significant, yet they do not affect a patient's quality of life; other times, the findings are absent or minimal, yet the patient experiences severe discomfort. For example, in arthritis it is common to find that the subjective experience of pain and disability is not linked to the structural changes seen on a radiograph. There are also times when objective measurements indicate disharmony, such as a routine blood work indicating diabetes, or blood pressure measurement indicating hypertension. In these situations, the goal of the practitioner is to look at other functional, structural, or psychological aspects of a patient to determine other ways that the body is mirroring that same pattern. For example, a patient may be unaware that their blood pressure is high, but they are aware that they are chronically constipated, that they have digestive problems, headaches, or that they are going through a tremendous amount of stress that they are internalizing (Lad 2005).

The total energy involved in the body is always constant, yet the amount of useful energy is diminished or dissipates as disease sets in (Capra 1988). In a health state, the energy moves freely. The wave patterns are in sync, are smooth, and display their normal amplitude and frequency. As disease sets in, the wave patterns change. The aspect of the patient that is overwhelmed or exhausted contracts or constricts, resulting in a change, and a disruption to the flow of energy to that area. As soon as any energy field constricts, the potential for healing in that area is limited. The aim of treatment is to understand a patient's pattern of response with the aim of intervening to expand their field – increase healing possibilities.

Transformation between health and disease

In a healthy state, human beings are able to adapt to and compensate for a wide range of factors all the time. When disturbing factors become too much for a patient, symptoms manifest on some level. 'Symptoms and signs are the only way we have of perceiving the workings of the defense mechanisms' (Vithoulkas 1981). After a patient recognizes the onset of symptoms they have options. They can respond to the symptoms in a way that restores health, they can acknowledge the symptoms and choose to palliate or suppress the symptoms, or they can ignore the symptoms. At every step of the process, a patient has the ability to make changes, to address the impact of the disturbance, and to restore health. If the symptoms are ignored, or the response to symptoms doesn't restore health, then one of two things usually happens. The frequency, intensity, or duration of the symptoms increases, or additional symptoms, on some level, start to appear, indicating a progressive breakdown of some other aspect of the patient.

Most people are dealing with many disrupting factors, in various degrees of severity and intensity, all the time. When the root causes of these factors are identified and addressed, it is possible for health to be restored. Along with the root cause, there often are aggravating factors that have a tendency to intensify or diminish the impact of the disruption. It is helpful, and sometimes necessary, to address the aggravating factors first as a means of lessening the impact that the root cause is having on a patient's health. If only the aggravating factors are treated then the signs and symptoms might be diminished, sometimes significantly, but true healing has not occurred and often the symptoms or a progression of the symptoms or disease will reappear. When true healing has occurred the key indicators to health will be strong, the need to support the body with supplements, herbs, medications or other treatments will be eliminated or dramatically reduced, and the signs and symptoms that indicated a disruption will be resolved. It is only by addressing the catalyst, the root cause of a disease, that the patient is able to return to harmony and health within the self.

Naturopathic medicine recognizes that the movement from health to disease is a two-way continuum, where the onset of symptoms does not necessarily mean the progression to disease. The challenge for a practitioner is to recognize and understand what the symptoms are conveying, that is, whether the presence of symptoms is an indication of a progression and worsening of a disease state, or whether they indicate that the body is attempting to heal and to reestablish health.

The stages of disease are similar for all three aspects of a patient – the psychological, the functional, and the structural. I encourage practitioners to be able to see, hear, and observe the stages of diseases in all aspects. The following section explores four types of transformation that occur: the acute healing response, a healing crisis, the immediate onset of disease, and the progression to chronic disease. Having an understanding of all four is essential to a practitioner working with and supporting the healing ability of the body.

Acute healing response

Acute states come on suddenly and are usually initiated by an exposure to an external pathogen or a minor injury, such as flus and colds, cutting your finger, eating spoiled food, coming in contact with poison ivy, bruising your leg, or falling and injuring yourself. 'Every acute disease is the result of a purifying, healing effort of nature' (Lindlahr 1975). The innate response of a patient, in these situations, is to initiate physiological responses to balance and harmonize the disturbing factors and to reestablish a homeodynamic state.

Acute symptoms, exhibiting the greatest vital response, usually take the form of inflammatory conditions, colds, influenza, diarrhea and rashes. Inflammation is described by Hans Seyle as an active defence reaction which is necessary to maintain health (Seyle 1978 in Turner 2000).

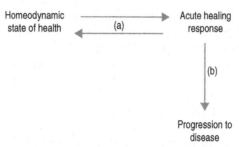

Fig 7.1 Acute healing response. An 'acute healing response' represents an individual's inherent ability to heal from sudden, disrupting factors such as external pathogens. (a) When the 'acute healing response' is supported health is restored. (b) When the 'acute healing response' is suppressed or when an individual is lacking the essential nutrients and qualities to support healing, health is disrupted at deeper levels.

During an acute healing response (Fig. 7.1) it is best to support the body, not to override it or suppress it. 'If a patient complains of one or more trivial symptoms that have been only observed a short time previously, the physician should not regard this as a fully developed disease that requires serious medical aid. A slight alternation in the diet and regimen will usually suffice to dispel such an indisposition (Hahnemann 1997). For example, a natural response to the flu is a fever and it is important to support this response, even to encourage it, and in doing so support the up-regulation of the immune system and the ability of the body to heal. Suppressing the fever, which is done all too often, weakens the immune system, hence making the patient more susceptible over time to infection (Kluger et al 1996).

During an acute healing response, the healing intention of the body focuses on the acute situation. If there is an underlying chronic condition, the healing will be partially suspended until the acute situation is addressed. For example, if a patient has chronic arthritis and then 'catches' a cold, the body naturally shifts the focus to resolving the cold. This response can be overridden by a patient's lifestyle or by taking medications or supplements that give the body a different message. For example, it is common to have a decreased appetite with a fever. The decrease in appetite is a message from the body that it is 'busy' healing. If a patient ignores this message and eats a large meal it diverts or shifts the body's focus, which results in slower healing or an impaired healing response.

When acute conditions are properly handled, the body returns to a homeodynamic state. If the acute response is suppressed or does not completely heal, the area of the body affected becomes weakened and more susceptible to injury or attack in the future. The continual suppression or lack of resolve of acute conditions results in a chronic disease condition.

A healing crisis

It is common for the body to initiate signs of healing as it moves from a disease state to one of health. 'A healing crisis is an acute, self-limiting, self-resolving symptom or set of symptoms' (Louise 2007). A 'healing crisis' is often a necessary part of the process of recovery (Turner 2000). The symptoms that arise during a healing crisis relate to those symptoms that were suppressed or unresolved. For example, if a patient has a history of asthma that has been suppressed, it would be common, and often desirable, for the patient to get an ear infection, as the respiratory and immune functions are strengthened. In a situation such as this, during the intake with the patient, the practitioner would have most likely discovered that as a child the patient had several ear infections that had been suppressed with antibiotics and other treatments.

The suppressed symptoms typically arise in reverse order, that is the symptoms that a patient experienced last manifest first in the healing process; ending with the symptoms that caused the initial episode.

> *Put very simply this means that many chronic diseases show a tendency to become worse before they get better; the more acute and superficial symptoms, if they were the first to appear, will usually be the last to go (Turner 2000).*

The presence of a healing crisis is a positive sign, as it indicates the strength of the body's healing potential. It is common for a naturopathic doctor to intentionally stimulate a healing crisis, such as hydrotherapy treatments to stimulate a fever. It is also important for a naturopathic doctor to educate their patients on the significance and potential of a healing crisis, as it is common for patients who are new to naturopathic medicine to mistake the healing crisis as a sign that their previous disease state is returning.

A healing crisis (Fig. 7.2) is an indication that the patient is returning to a greater state of health. As such, when a healing crisis occurs, the other indicators of health and vitality are typically stronger – such as sleep, appetite, energy level, mental outlook, blood results, tongue and pulse diagnosis, and skin color. During a healing crisis, it is important to support the body and allow it to properly deal with the underlying imbalance. The more that the building blocks to health are addressed, and adhered to, the less aggravating the healing crisis usually is to the patient.

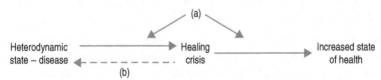

Fig 7.2 Healing crisis. A healing crisis indicates a movement from a disease state to a higher state of health. (a) When the healing crisis is supported the patient enjoys an increased state of health. (b) If the healing crisis is suppressed or incomplete the disease process continues to progress.

Immediate onset of disease

Mild and moderate disturbing factors initiate the acute healing response, but when the exposure to an infectious agent, external factor, or significant event is extreme, it results in a more dramatic impact to health and the immediate onset of disease. The aspect of the patient affected and the degree of the impact depends on the disturbing factor. The following are examples of an immediate onset of disease: the onset of extreme anxiety and intense chest pains after hearing that a loved one has died unexpectedly; major bleeding or fractures due to a motor vehicle accident; or severe nausea and gastric bleeding after ingesting a poison.

The impact of specific events, situations, and external factors depends partly on the level of a patient's health at the time that the disturbing factor 'hit'. For example, if a patient is in a homeostatic state, that is they are healthy, they will recover more easily from an accident than a patient who is already dealing with degenerative changes in their health. Immediate threats, if they are not treated appropriately, often progress to more severe diseases or risks to health quickly. The treatment strategy often involves the use of therapeutic agents, and/or medical interventions.

Progression to chronic disease

When mild symptoms are not addressed or resolved, a worsening of the symptoms often occurs, resulting eventually in chronic disease. Chronic disease is the result of prolonged and continual disruption in the needed resources for health. Loeser & Melzack (1999) looked at chronic pain and in their findings they suggest that it is not the duration of pain that distinguishes acute from chronic, but the inability of the body to restore its physiological functions to normal homeodynamic levels.

The timing and progression of disease depends on a number of factors that are continuously at play, such as a patient's constitution, their susceptibilities, their adherence to the building blocks of health, and their exposure to external and environment disrupting factors. The onset of chronic disease is influenced by the manner in which a patient addresses and handles signs and symptoms throughout their life, and it depends on the severity and impact of any particular disrupting factor.

> Chronic disease never develops suddenly in the human body. Nature always tries to prevent its gradual development by acute and subacute healing efforts. If these, by any means whatever, are checked and suppressed, then they are followed either by fatal complications or chronic after effects, the mysterious 'sequelae' of medical science (Lindlahr 1975).

Most holistic medical systems recognize that disease is a progressive process (Fig. 7.3) and that this process, for the most part, has the ability to move in both directions. Understanding the stages helps a practitioner to know how to 'unwind' the disease process and to move from a chronic state back to health. The following is an overview of the progression of a chronic disease. The initial stages have symptoms that are more excretory and that appear in the more superficial areas of the body. Over time, as disease progresses, the symptoms become deeper and more internal. This coincides with the Yin–Yang theory that acute diseases are more Yang in nature, and chronic diseases are more Yin.

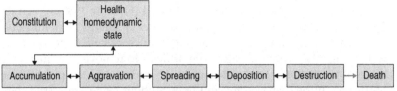

Fig 7.3 Progressive stages of disease. The accumulation of excesses and deficiencies in a person's lifestyle and in their environment leads to progressive deterioration in health. Symptoms of aggravation spread to other aspects and the continual presence of disrupting factors leads to the deposition or crystallization of energy. This deposition affects the flow of energy and leads to destruction of the structure, function, or psychological aspects and eventually results in death.

1. *Constitution.* Constitutional qualities dictate a patient's strength, areas of susceptibility, vitality, and their uniqueness; it represents the baseline line or health that a patient was born with. The beginning section of this chapter explores constitution in more detail.

2. *Health – homeodynamic state.* In an aim to maintain health, a patient is continuously accommodating, compensating for, and adapting to different internal and external factors. Homeodynamics is a process of self-regulation, and self-renewal.

3. *Accumulation.* When a patient can no longer adapt and compensate for the disrupting factors, symptoms result (Frawley 1989). The initial symptoms often involve an excretory reaction and result in symptoms such as irritation or inflammation, sweating, fever, diarrhea, or acute muscle pain or weakness, or psychological disturbances such as mild anxiety frustration. The aspect of accumulation relates to the patient's constitution, areas of susceptibility, and the characteristics of the disrupting factors.

4. *Aggravation.* As the excesses build at a greater degree than they are excreted or balanced, the signs and symptoms of disharmony become more intense and more constant. As the quality of one part or organ system of the body becomes exaggerated, it will result in the depletion of another and the hyperactivity of other parts (Beinfield & Korngold 1991). Aggravation manifests in symptoms such as chronic inflammation, continual stiffness, chronic pain, or intense thoughts, depending on the aspect of the individual that is aggravated. At this stage, symptoms are still relatively easy to remove by addressing the initiating and aggravating factors, and improving the building blocks to health.

5. *Spreading.* All organ systems and aspects of the body are a network, where one part feeds and nurtures another part. When a specific organ or part of a patient reaches its threshold, the aggravation spills over into other parts. The area of spread depends on a patient's constitution and the nature of the factors that overwhelmed the patient. For example, if the digestive tract is overloaded it might spread to the skin or to the joints. If the kidneys are overloaded, you might find symptoms of pain or peripheral swelling. The symptoms are still relatively easy to clear at this stage.

6. *Deposition.* If the appropriate steps are not taken to address the signs and symptoms of spreading, the symptoms will become more ingrained in the body. The patterns become more fixed and 'sit' in the areas of

susceptibility or in the areas that are affected (Frawley 1989). When the energy 'sits' in an area it will result in a block of energy flow into that area, resulting in symptoms such as fatty tissues, calculi, nodes, and cysts. At this stage the symptoms are more difficult to remove. It requires more intervention and attention on behalf of the patient and the practitioner.

7. *Destruction.* If the disharmony continues without being addressed the tissues or functions involved eventually start to deteriorate and break down and there is destruction in function and in structure. This area often is associated with conditions such as cancer, cirrhosis, and organ failure. At this stage there often is a definable disease, and the disease and the symptoms often are difficult to remove. This stage requires intervention on many different levels. As an individual becomes overwhelmed and exhausted, the pattern shifts to a deficiency state, even if the overall disrupting factors were due to excesses.

8. *Death.* Eventually the progression of disease leads to death. The rate of progression and the symptoms associated with the progression depend on a number of different factors, and on the mind-set of the patient.

The manifestation of chronic disease is unique for everyone. Once disease has been established it takes on a life of its own. Patients are complex systems that have encountered very different experiences and variables in their lives. This uniqueness influences the manifestation of disease and the impact that any disease has on a patient. By understanding where disease is in its evolution it allows a practitioner to direct the type of treatment that is used.

ASPECTS OF MANIFESTATION

The strength of each aspect – psychological, functional or structural – of a patient is reflected in its ability to resist disease. It is determined by a patient's constitution and vitality, their attention to the building blocks to health, and their exposure to disrupting external and environmental factors. All aspects manifest disease, and disease affects all aspects at once. The aspect that is the 'loudest' – often the one that demonstrates the greatest degree of shift – corresponds to the disturbing factor that initiated the shift from health. If the impact of the symptoms continues for a long period of time, without resolution or addressing the disrupting factors, there is a greater chance that the impact on the functional and structural aspects will show greater signs of deterioration, as they are denser forms of energy.

Primary site of manifestation

The primary site is where the impact first 'hit'; the aspect of the patient that is the most affected by the initial stimulus. For example, if you fall playing sports, the structural aspect of the body – such as a knee injury – will be the primary site. If you are concerned about giving a speech, the psychological aspect – such as a feeling of anxiety – will be the primary site. If you are sick because of eating too much food it will primarily affect the functional aspect – resulting in symptoms such as diarrhea, stomach pain, or nausea and vomiting.

Secondary sites of manifestation

All symptoms, to varying degrees, impact all three levels at once (Fig. 7.4). If the psychological aspect is the primary site, the functional and structural will be secondary; and so on. For example, in the case of a sports injury, the structural aspect – the knee – is the primary site; secondarily, on a psychological level a patient might experience disappointment, anger, or frustration, depending on how the injury happened and what the injury means to them; on a functional level, the injury might result in inflammation, nerve damage, or muscular changes.

Sometimes the secondary symptoms are what a patient notes as their chief complaint. For example, a patient who is anxious might be concerned with his shortness of breath or heart palpitations, not recognizing that the symptoms are due to a psychological state. A patient might be concerned with leg pain that is actually being caused by an ovarian cyst. Because all aspects of a patient are interrelated, it is possible to influence many health concerns by working with the secondary sites of manifestation. For example, teaching patients how to breathe effectively (a functional activity) has been proven to be an effective treatment for anxiety (a psychological activity) (Chow & Tsang 2007, Lolak et al 2008). Addressing posture and physical alignment (which is structural work) can be an effective way of improving digestive function (Asada et al 1989, Hirota et al 2002).

It is important for a practitioner to recognize whether symptoms are primary or secondary. If only the symptoms in the secondary sites are treated, the treatment might be unsuccessful, especially if the disrupting factor is still present and sending a message of disharmony to the primary site. On the other hand, when the secondary sites of manifestation are addressed, a patient might experience relief and improvement in their overall quality and life, thus providing patients with the motivation, energy, or ability to

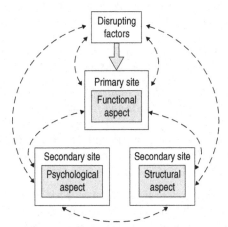

Fig 7.4 Impact of symptoms. When disrupting factors cause a state of overwhelm, symptoms impact all three aspects of an individual – psychological, functional, and structural – at once. The primary site of impact represents the aspect of an individual that was most affected by the disrupting factor. If the functional is the primary site, the psychological and structural will be secondary. Likewise, if the primary site is the psychological the secondary sites will be the functional and structural – and so on. All parts interact with each other and are influenced by each other.

Health and disease

address the disrupting factors that are causing the symptoms on the primary site. On the other hand, some patients, when they feel better, do not pursue their healing process further; there is a sense of 'I feel fine so why should I continue treatment.'

Psychological level

Changes that affect primarily the *psychological* level occur when a patient's life is misaligned with their personal essence, when there is a disruption on the social level, or when a stressful event or situation has happened. The psychological aspect is the primary site of signs and symptoms when there is a sense of discontentment with an aspect of one's life, or when there is a sense of being overwhelmed with external commitments and responsibilities, or an inability to express oneself.

When an event happens that 'triggers' a patient, that is it affects them deeply, the conscious mind is activated. There is mental awareness either of the event, the consequences, or both. The response to an event depends on a patient's constitution, their fears, beliefs, cumulative life experiences, and the current state of their health. For example, a patient who is confident and believes that 'all feedback is good feedback' is likely to respond positively if a boss recommends areas that he needs to improve upon; if, on the other hand, he has a weaker sense of self, and believes that 'he needs to be perfect', he is more likely to respond negatively to the same feedback. Most people will have an opinion about or an emotional response to such an event. At any point in time during the process, the patient can adjust their thoughts or 'work through' an event and restore a healthy balance in the body. When the event stays 'negatively charged' the impact progresses and the patient shifts further away from health.

Disharmony, in the psychological aspect, manifests as intensity in thoughts or emotions; such as doubt, worry, fear, anger, or jealousy. Psychological disruptions are mirrored in functional changes, such as posture, breathing, heart rate, digestion or sleep. People who are stubborn and rigid in their mental attitude (an earth quality) are usually physically tight and stiff (also earth qualities) (Mattsson & Mattsson 2002).

> Research at the Institute for Heart Math (McCraty et al 2001) has shown a relationship between emotional state and frequency spectrum of the electrical signals from the heart. Feelings of love, caring and compassion, or of frustration and anger, will affect the signals produced by the heart. These signals are conducted to every cell in the body and are radiated into the space around the body (Oshman 2003).

> Emotions are inseparable from the simultaneous bodily changes. The slightest alterations of the emotional balance are registered instantly as a change in the biophysical and biochemical state of the body (Thass-Theinemann 1968).

Often, when there is freedom in expression, the disrupting factors result in less functional or structural changes, especially over time. When the psychological level is in a state of harmony and contentment, it can improve the healing ability of the patient; when it is in a fear state or in disharmony, it can impede the body's ability to heal.

The psychological level is considered the secondary site when it manifests disruption in response to changes on the functional or structural level. Examples are frustration over cutting your finger, fear associated with an asthmatic attack, or feeling of weakness due to poor posture or muscle pain.

Functional level

The *functional* level is the primary area to shift when the cause of disease is due to imbalances in breathing, food, fluid, sleep, and rest, and when the body has been dealing with an excess and deficiency in diet, or nutritional disruptors, or toxins for a long time. This level often is associated with chronic diseases, either as a causal or an aggravating factor.

The body has a tremendous ability to compensate and adapt to functional variances in the body, based on changing internal and external influences. Each cell structure and metabolic capability dictates the amount of physiological demand it can handle. The homeodynamic state of cellular function is maintained when the physiological demands do not surpass the metabolic capabilities.

Cells can alter their functional state in response to modest stress and maintain their homeostasis. They react to more excessive physiological stresses, or adverse pathologic stimuli, by (1) adapting, (2) sustaining reversible injury, or (3) suffering irreversible injury and dying (Robbins & Cotran 1999).

The body starts to display functional changes on the cellular and chemical level as the impact of the disrupting factors becomes more than the body can handle. Functional changes manifest as a change in the chemical balance of blood, urine, or saliva, the tissues start to break down, the production of digestive juices, enzymes, hormones, and neurotransmitters becomes impeded, or there is a build up of toxins in the body, inflammation and an accumulation of waste products. Typically, there is a disruption in the flow of nutrients and energy across the cellular membranes, a blockage in the body's ability to eliminate toxins, or a change in the flow of emotions.

The functional level impacts both the psychological and the structural levels. It is considered a secondary site when changes are due to disruptions in the level of the psychological or structural; such as structural changes that impede proper breathing or constipation due to chronic worrying. When the functional level is in a state of deficiency or excess, such as in the case of nutrient deficiency, lack of water consumption, or lack of proper breathing; it results in changes on the psychological and structural aspects. For example, a deficiency in nutrients or sleep might result in an increase in anxiety or irritability, a patient 'has a shorter fuse' and reacts to situations that they usually are okay with. A patient with improper breathing often ends up with structural changes in their upper torso.

Health and disease

Structural level

Signs and symptoms often manifest on the *structural* level when they are a result of posture, ergonomics, exercise or movement, accident or injury. When the injuries and accidents are acute there is typically an awareness of the specific cause, such as a car accident, sports injury or fall. In acute situations it is important to identify if there is a weakness in the underlying aspects that is making the structure more susceptible, especially if the injury occurs more than once; for example, if a patient repeatedly and easily injures their shoulder.

Structural changes accompany changes in the psychological and in the functional. If you think about being strong, confident, and successful, you notice your body straighten and breathing become deeper. When you feel like withdrawing from others, feeling depressed or weak, your body contracts and breathing becomes shallower. As a patient's state of health deteriorates, their structure, both at the cellular and the physical level, will change.

REFERENCES

Asada T, Sako Y, Fukushima Y, Kita T, Miyake T 1989 Effect of body position on gastric emptying of solid food – a study using a sulfamethizole capsule food method. Japn J Gastro-Enterol 86(8): 1604–1610

Baron RJ 1985 An introduction to medical phenomenology: I can't hear you while I'm listening. Ann Intern Med 103: 606–611

Beinfield H, Korngold E 1991 Between Heaven and Earth, a Guide to Chinese Medicine. Ballantine Wellspring, New York

Capra F 1988 The Turning Point, science, society, and the rising culture. Bantam Books, Toronto

Chow YW, Tsang HW 2007 Biopsychosocial effects of Qigong as a mindful exercise for people with anxiety disorders: a speculative review. J Altern Complement Med 13(8):831–839

Duffin J 2007 History of Medicine. University of Toronto Press, Toronto

Frawley D 1989 Ayurvedic Healing, a Comprehensive Guide. Salt Lake City, Utah

Hahnemann S 1997 Organon of Medicine, sixth Edition. B. Jain Publishers, New Delhi

Hirota N, Sone Y, Tokura H 2002 Effect of postprandial posture on digestion and absorption of dietary carbohydrate. J Physiol Anthropol Appl Hum Sci 21(1):45–50

Idler EL, Kasl S 1991 Health perceptions and survival: Do global evaluations of health status really predict mortality? J Gerontol 46:55

Justice B 1998 Being well inside the self: A different measure of health. Advances in Mind-Body Medicine 14(1):61–68

Kluger MJ, Kozak W, Conn CA, Leon LR, Soszynski D 1996 The adaptive value of fever. Infect Dis Clin N Am 10(1):1–20

Lad V 1998 Ayurveda, the Science of Self-healing. Lotus Light Publications, Delhi

Lad V 2005 Ayurvedic Perspectives on Selected Pathologies. The Ayurvedic Press, New Mexico

Lindlahr H 1975 Philosophy of Natural Therapeutics. CW Daniel Company, England

Lipton B 2005 The Biology of Belief, Unleashing the Power of Consciousness Matter & Miracles. Elite Books, California

Loeser JD, Melzack R 1999 Pain: an overview. Lancet 353:1607–1609

Lolak S, Connors GL, Sheridan MJ, Wise TN 2008 Effects of progressive muscle relaxation training on anxiety and depression in patients enrolled in an outpatient pulmonary rehabilitation program. Psychother Psychosom 77(2):119–125

Louise C 2007 Systems Principles and Naturopathic Philosophy: The Human Being as a Complex System. Presented at the First International Editors Retreat, Foundations of Naturopathic Medicine Project

Maciocia G 1989 The Foundations of Chinese Medicine. Churchill Livingstone, Edinburgh

Mattsson B, Mattsson M 2002 The concept of 'psychosomatic' in general practice. Reflections on body language and a tentative model for understanding. Scand J Prim Health Care 20(1):135–138

McCraty R, Atkinson M, Tomasino D 2001 The electricity of touch: detection and measurement of cardiac energy exchange between people. In Oshman J 2003 Energy Medicine in Therapeutics and Human Performance. Butterworth-Heinemann, Edinburgh

McTaggart L 2002 The Field, the Quest for the Secret Force of the Universe. Harper Collins, London

Mitchell B 2007 The Vis Part 1 and 2. Presented at the First International Editors Retreat, Foundations of Naturopathic Medicine Project

Murray MT, Pizzorno JE 1991 Encyclopedia of Natural Medicine. Prima Publishing, California

Oschman J 2003 Energy Medicine in Therapeutics and Human Performance. Butterworth-Heinemann, Edinburgh

Robbins SL, Cotran RS et al (eds) 1999 Pocket Companion to Robbins Pathological Basis of Disease, sixth edition. WB Saunders, Philadelphia

Roehrs T, Roth T 2008 Caffeine: sleep and daytime sleepiness. Sleep Med Rev 12(2):153–162

Svoboda RE 1989 Prakruti, your Ayurvedic Constitution. Lotus Press, New Mexico

Thass-Thienemann T 1968 Symbolic Behavior. Washington Square Press, New York

Turner RN 2000 Naturopathic Medicine, Treating the Whole Patient. Thorsons, UK

Vithoulkas G 1981 The Science of Homeopathy. Grove Press, New York

FURTHER READING

Bickley LS, Hoekelman RA 1999 Physical Examination and History Taking, seventh edition. Lippincott, Philadelphia

Brotman DJ, Golden SH, Wittstein IS 2007 The cardiovascular tool of stress. Lancet 370:1089–1100.

Fosha D 2006 Quantum Transformation in trauma and treatment: traversing the crisis of healing change. J Clin Psychol 62(5):569–583

Lindlahr H 1985 Iridiagnosis and other diagnostic methods, Natural Therapeutics Vol. 4. Hillman Printers, UK

Lloyd IR 2005 Messages from the Body, a Guide to the Energetics of Health. Naturopathic Publications, Toronto

Magner LN 1992 A History of Medicine. Marcel Dekker, New York

Penson RT, Partridge RA, Shah MA, Giansiracusa D, Chabner BA, Lynch TJ Jr 2005 Fear of death. Oncologist 10(2):160–169

Penson RT, Gu F, Harris S, et al 2007 Hope. Oncologist 12:1105–1113

Pole S 2006 Ayurvedic Medicine, the Principles of Traditional Practice. Elsevier, Philadelphia

Zeff JL 1997 The process of healing: a unifying theory of naturopathic medicine. J Naturopath Med 7(1):122

Health and disease

SECTION III
NATUROPATHIC ASSESSMENT

CHAPTER 8
The therapeutic encounter

With a holistic approach to health and disease the importance of the therapeutic encounter is paramount. During an assessment a practitioner considers the spiritual, psychological, functional, and structural aspects of a patient. They inquire about the building blocks to health, family, social, environmental, and external factors. A thorough assessment includes the current physiological and pathological state of a patient. The aim is to identify the initiating and aggravating factors that are contributing to the symptoms and illness, and to determine what needs to change or what a patient requires in order to stimulate their innate healing ability and to achieve a desired state of wellness. Subsequent visits assist with understanding how a patient is progressing on their journey to health and in identifying new patterns as they emerge.

It is through the verbal part of the assessment that the initiating and aggravating factors are uncovered. The symptoms reveal 'what' is going on, but only by talking to the patient, is the 'why' uncovered. It is the 'why' that is key to determining what changes are required and what treatment is appropriate and needed. A practitioner then correlates the patterns associated with the subjective symptoms with the patterns that emerge thorough a physical exam. Naturopathic doctors utilize the knowledge gained by blood tests, radiographs, scans, and other objective measurements, but they place a high value on a patient's subjective experiences and the information that can be obtained from the patient, such as tongue and pulse diagnosis, looking at the alignment of specific aspects of the body, and mapping the manifestation of symptoms to the energetics of particular body parts.

The inquiry into the cause of symptoms and diseases and how to detect illness in the body has always been at the heart of the medical profession. The methods used for assessment have changed substantially over time, and prior to the eighteenth century, history taking and diagnosing was based on the subjective symptoms of patients (Magner 1992). As the conventional medical field introduced more objective means of assessing health and disease, the relationship between the patient and the practitioner became more distant. The information obtained by objective measures was, and often is, taken as more valuable than the subjective information conveyed by a patient. In a naturopathic and holistic assessment a practitioner must value and integrate both the subjective symptoms and the objective signs, and recognize that the patient is more important than the disease. 'In other words, the subjective should be part of a disease, just as it is part of being ill. If we find a way to include the subjective in our concepts of disease, maybe we will also discover purpose and meaning' (Duffin 2007).

The naturopathic approach is based on the understanding that health and disease are multi-factorial and that there is a logical pattern that links the patient's behavior and symptoms with their lifestyle, environment, and external factors (Fig. 8.1). This pattern emerges when we see all aspects of life and nature from the perspective of their qualities and attributes. During the therapeutic encounter a practitioner is looking at putting all the pieces together and determining the overall patterns for each patient. It is by treating the patterns and the patient as an integrated whole that health is achieved and maintained.

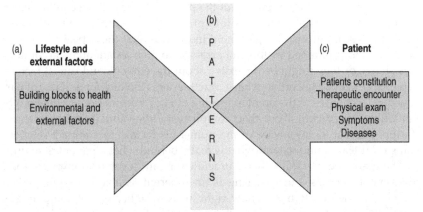

Fig 8.1 Patterns as the common factor. (a) Lifestyle and external factors – all factors can be broken down and understood based on their specific patterns. (b) Patterns – relate to the qualities and attributes, such as internal/external Yin Yang, excess/deficiency, and the five elements. (c) Patient – all aspects of a patient carry and manifest the same patterns.

PATIENT–PRACTITIONER RELATIONSHIP

Communication, both verbal and non-verbal, is the medium through which relationships begin and develop. The *quality* of communication directly influences the *quality* of the relationship and it is strongly linked to patient adherence and satisfaction (Bernstein & Bernstein 1985, Barrier et al 2003, Platt & Gordon 2004). The primary purpose of the patient–practitioner relationship is the optimal well-being of the patient. The reason for the initial visit is for the patient to convey to the practitioner their medical history and to provide the practitioner with a window into who they are and how they live their life. The therapeutic encounter is not simply an exchange of information; it is, or can be, therapeutic in and of itself. A detailed and attentive intake often is the first time that many patients have been able to convey 'their story' and feel heard. The ability of a practitioner to hear the correlation between a patient's complaints and their constitution, or situations that have happened in a patient's life and their symptoms is a valuable skill. Occasionally, a patient might even experience extraordinary 'spontaneous' healings of very serious injuries or diseases when there is a strong connection between the patient and practitioner (Murphy 1993).

As a guide and teacher, the naturopathic doctor is seen to provide a patient with a road map, and a list of changes and options to improve their well-being. The naturopathic medical philosophy, 'doctor as teacher' involves providing patients with a framework and understanding for health and disease. This is often done by teaching patients how to become aware of how their lifestyle aggravates or ameliorates their symptoms. The relationship is not about blind obedience or dependency, but involves the practitioner having the knowledge and skill to teach the patient how to live their life in a more harmonic way based on their unique characteristics. It also involves a practitioner having the skills, tools, and the knowledge of therapeutic substances to assist the body in restoring health and wellness.

The patient–practitioner relationship is influenced by the beliefs of the practitioner, the time and attention that each dedicates to the relationship, by the expectations and openness of the patient, and by the encounter itself. There are many factors that come into play. A practitioner might intimidate the patient or might convey judgment in the way that they speak. A patient might be too frightened or too embarrassed to give an adequate account of symptoms, or they might be defensive about the etiology and causal factors. A patient might be uncertain what a practitioner is looking for and might narrow their responses to the point of leaving out key information, or they might not tell the exact truth about their compliance if they anticipate judgment or disappointment. Being aware of the numerous factors that impact relationships is critical to understand what is really behind what a patient is saying.

There are specific skills that a practitioner can develop to improve their assessment abilities, but assessing is an inherent skill in everyone. When we meet a friend, often we know right away whether or not something is wrong. We avoid some people and gravitate to others based on their energy. We change our mind because things do not feel right. When you need assistance there is a reason why you choose to ask someone for help and not someone else. Interpreting the patterns of symptoms and diseases requires slowing down this inherent assessment process and paying attention to the details. It requires that a practitioner recognize the energetic qualities and attributes of all aspects of life and diseases. As a naturopathic doctor notices, tunes in to the details, and understands what the subtleness of the emerging patterns convey, they understand how an individual shifts in response to stress and trauma, and they can marvel at its ability to shift back.

Most patients are accustomed to having a very short time to convey their symptoms and their story to their general practitioner. When a visit with a patient is short or rushed it can greatly hamper the value of the therapeutic encounter.

From the point of view of the patient, then, the most serious barriers to a good relationship (and consequently better diagnosis and treatment) are the professional's lack of time, seeming lack of concern, and failure to tell the patient what the patient needs to know and can understand about the illness (Bernstein & Bernstein 1985).

Research also shows that spending time early in patient encounters saves time in the long run (Platt & Gordon 2004).

An initial intake with a naturopathic doctor is usually one to two hours in length, with follow-up visits typically 30 minutes in length. This time is essential for patients not only to convey their symptoms, but to relay their lifestyle patterns, to talk about the significant events that have occurred in their life, and to discuss their goals and intentions, and their beliefs about health and disease. The role of the practitioner is to listen to all the pieces of information and how they are communicated, and then put it all together in a way that makes sense and that gives direction and rationalization to a treatment strategy that accomplishes the patient's goals. Learning how to achieve and maintain wellness is an ongoing journey. Maintaining a strong therapeutic alliance requires the ongoing attention to the patient's subjective experiences of their life and their healing journey.

A naturopathic assessment links the symptom patterns to factors that have contributed to their onset. At times, the symbolic meaning of a single symptom 'jumps out'; when this happens it is important to avoid treating symptomatically or treating individual findings. What a practitioner is looking for is the underlying pattern, what ties all the symptoms together. You are looking for the factor or factors that initiated and contributed to the state of overwhelm and disharmony. For example, a patient might have a swollen left ankle because of collapsed veins, inability to hold her urine, spotting with her period, and rounded shoulders. The common thread, or pattern, is a lack of earth. There isn't enough earth for the vessels to hold in the blood or the lymphatic fluid, the bladder is lacking the strength to hold in the urine, and her structure is becoming rounded because of a lack of earth. The next step is to find out what has happened in her life to affect her earth; her sense of structure and support. For example, it could be when she lost her job all of a sudden, or when her marriage broke down, or it might be a life-long concern because she has always had a weak sense of confidence.

An understanding of the initiating and aggravating factors can seldom be made on one symptom. And not all things that you notice about a patient indicate a heterogenic or disease state. For example, there is a difference between a person who naturally has a broader right side, indicating a more naturally Yang disposition, and someone whose right side has expanded due to a life that is too Yang. In the first example, you will not find other symptoms of overwhelm due to Yang excess. In the second example, there will be other shifts, such as increased aggression, a red tongue with a thick yellow coat, arms that are held further from the body, or a red rash that is worse on the right arm.

Role of the practitioner

A practitioner is a guide and a facilitator of health. Their role is to listen and observe from a neutral place, without judgment or preconceived ideas. They use their skills and knowledge to identify the root cause of disease, and to provide the education and support that is needed for healing. To recognize the uniqueness of patients, to identify and remove obstacles to cure, to support the inherent healing ability of each patient, to recognize the stages of disease, and to prioritize treatment recommendations to ensure optimal wellness and a logical healing process. It is to be curious about health and to remember that health and disease have a logical pattern, to continually search for the truth and the factors that are at play for each individual patient. The aim of a practitioner is to translate the patterns back to the patient in a way that provides them with the knowledge to change what needs to be changed in order to restore wellness and a homeodynamic state. 'The most important treatment any doctor can give is to hope for the health and well being of his or her patients' (McTaggart 2002).

Another role of naturopathic practitioners is to recognize the difference in healing intentions and to understand and communicate to patients the difference between short-term treatment relief and long-term health strategies. There are many different windows that a practitioner can use for assessments and each practitioner has specific skills and attributes that increase their tendency to utilize one or more of the windows. For example, some practitioners are gifted at picking up information by listening to patients, other practitioners can tell a lot about a patient by pulse and tongue assessment, and others are skilled at reading the alignment of tissues and structures.

The specific energetic constitution and beliefs of a practitioner also impacts their approach and style with patients. It is valuable for practitioners to understand their own constitution, to recognize how they process information, and what their strengths and weaknesses are. For example, if a practitioner has a lot of 'earth' qualities, that is they are good at details and like order and continuity, they are more likely to get impatient with patients that are more scattered or that tend to go and on and on when speaking.

It is valuable for practitioners to continually clarify their own personal intentions and to ensure that they recognize that their role is to provide patients with choices and knowledge, not to 'fix them'. Sometimes the expectations of the practitioner and their need to help people can cloud their perspective on what is best for a patient. The challenge of transference and counter-transference comes into play. Recognizing the complexity of the therapeutic encounter, continually assessing intentions, and reviewing challenging situations with peers and professionals is continually needed as a medical practitioner.

Role of the patient

The role of the patient is integral to a successful therapeutic relationship. In order for a practitioner to utilize their skill, a patient needs to be forthcoming with key information. The more that a patient is aware of the nature of their symptoms, of what aggravates and what ameliorates them, the better a practitioner can understand the energetic patterns that are currently manifesting.

Assessment is not a guessing game, it is like a puzzle, and a practitioner needs as many pieces of the puzzle as possible. This involves recording a complete list of medications, supplements, and homeopathic remedies; other treatments, including dental, cosmetic, and energetic; an understanding of external factors, which might include the type of cooking utensils, how a patient's house is heated, the use of microwave ovens, cell phones, etc. What often is surprising to a patient is the breadth and depth of inquiry in a naturopathic assessment. As practitioners and patients recognize the growing number of factors that impact health, the role of the patient becomes more extensive, as they are the ones that can confirm the exposure to individual factors and the impact that key factors have had.

THE HOLISTIC INTAKE

I have chosen to use the term 'holistic intake' instead of history taking due to the breadth of the intake. A holistic intake includes the medical history of the patient, their family history, an overview of their lifestyle, social history, a review of environmental factors and other external factors that impact the patient's life. It also includes understanding the patient's goals and beliefs about their illness, their health and their potential to heal.

The importance of the history cannot be overestimated. Studies performed with hospital out-patients show that diagnoses are made from the history in the vast majority of patients. Examinations only provide significant unexpected findings in a minority (Welsby 2002).

Every encounter with a patient, whether the first time or follow up, involves conversation. The conversation is an integral part of the ongoing assessment process and it requires time and attention. It is through conversation that a patient can tell their story, that they can indicate the impact that their life has had on them, and their desire for change. Conducting a thorough history is not unique to naturopathic medicine. The difference is that a naturopathic practitioner typically asks a broader range of questions and asks for more details on each component of the intake. A holistic intake explores the following:

- the essence of who the patient is
- how the patient perceives health and disease
- what a patient thinks about their life
- what the patient wants or expects from the practitioner
- how the patient experiences their symptoms and illness and what impact it has on their life
- what aggravates or ameliorates the symptoms and the specifics on the nature of the symptoms
- the associated symptoms and their timing of onset
- the patient's ideas and feelings about their illness and their ability to heal
- to what degree a patient sees the correlation between their lifestyle and their symptoms
- their family and medical history
- the situations or events in a patient's life that are have impacted them
- the external and environmental factors that impact a patient's life

Conversation is important to build rapport between the patient and the practitioner, and it keeps the patient actively involved in the therapeutic encounter. Determining *what* the body is expressing is not the difficult or critical aspect of an assessment, it is determining *why* the body is expressing and holding a specific pattern that is important. The answers lie within the patient and come from the conversation. Through this conversation, a practitioner is able to assist their patient in hearing and seeing how their symptoms relate to their life, and to situations that have happened. When a patient comes in to see a practitioner inquiring about a specific symptom or disease state, the role of the practitioner is to recognize that the map differs from the territory. For example, when a patient comes in with a flare up of psoriasis (the territory) a practitioner would ask about the history (the map) that got them there.

History taking includes listening, questioning and observation. It recognizes the impact and significance of words and realizes that patients reveal how their life and their symptoms relate; if a practitioner just takes the time and learns how to truly listen. There are many good books written on history taking skills. The purpose of this book is to introduce the concepts of energetic patterns, as they are conveyed in a history taking.

PATTERNS CONVEYED THROUGH LANGUAGE

Words and language are powerful. They can stimulate the healing process or block it. The words that patients use, and the words that practitioners use, have a direct and dramatic impact on the therapeutic encounter. Words trigger memories and they are used as a way of tracking, labeling, and categorizing our experiences.

It is of inestimable importance that we are able to listen deeply to our patient's words and to be aware of our own. The quality of our ability to think deeply and consistently about the unconscious experience of our patient is intimately related to our ability to hear what is being said. The effect of our own words upon the patient likewise cannot be overstated (Proner 2006).

The words that a patient uses describe the qualities and the subjective experience of symptoms. Patients use words such as, wet, dry, hot, cold, rough, smooth, constricted, heavy, stiff, blocked, weak, etc. These terms can also be used to describe the qualities of foods, behaviors, and situations. The words often mirror the patterns or behaviors that caused the symptoms. By listening to a patient's words a practitioner will be guided to the underlying patterns that are causing the disruption to health.

The structure of language reflects a patient's mental organization, their unconscious perceptions, and their beliefs. The conscious and unconscious create expectations and boundaries and convey a patient's perceived limitations, not actual limitations. How a patient speaks and what they say, both outwardly and internally, provides a road map that explains how they have interpreted events in their past, how they see the present, and their outlook on the future.

If a patient cannot envision being well it is unlikely they will achieve wellness; as their mind is capable of overriding the healing process. There are also times when a patient conveys that they 'feel better than they thought possible'. When this happens it is important to recognize the significance of these words and to assist patients in increasing their expectations and in recognizing that they might have more healing potential than they initially realized.

Meaning of words

The meaning of each word is complex and unique to that patient. Words are symbolic triggers that have energy and that bring into consciousness aspects of a patient's experience (Bandler & Grinder 1979). Speech is a form of symbolic behavior and it holds meaning.

Thought processes suppose context and meaning. One cannot simply think; one has to think something. One does not simply 'behave,' but behavior is directed toward a conscious or unconscious goal (Thass-Theinemann 1968).

A patient's choice of language is unconscious to a large degree and reflects the energy within. It reflects the depth of the shift in the body, the willingness and vitality of a patient to heal, and a patient's expectations and beliefs. For example, patients use phrases such as:

- 'It can't be cured.'
- 'It is a progressive disease.'
- 'I guess I'm just getting old.'
- 'I know I'll always be on medication.'
- 'I am just looking for the pain to decrease so that it is more bearable.'
- 'I could get by even if I had a couple of good nights of sleep a week.'
- 'I would like better control of my blood pressure.'

There is a difference between a patient looking to manage their pain better and having the expectation and belief that they can be pain free; or a patient expecting that it is normal to have a good night's sleep every night, instead of just once in awhile; or a patient believing that once they have hypertension they will have it for ever. In order for a patient to change their perception and way that they interpret events in their life, they need to bring their unconscious beliefs and expectations to their consciousness (Murphy 1993). If a patient has a limiting belief about their symptoms or state of disease, it limits the degree of health that they achieve.

The language that is spoken everyday which is more subtle and repetitive affects health at a deeper level. Most people are unaware of how they reinforce internal patterns solely based on their language. Words carry an energetic pattern, a message to the rest of the body. If that message continually is that a person needs to be 'on guard' or that they 'aren't safe' the functional and structural aspects of the body respond accordingly, by constricting components of the body or blocking the flow of energy to an area.

Limiting beliefs

When practitioners have limited beliefs about the healing power of the body, and the logic of health and disease, they 'train' patients to believe certain things. For example, it is common for a conventionally trained medical practitioner to belief that once a patient has hypertension and is put on medication they will be on it for the rest of their life. But what if the hypertension is primarily due to a separation or a loss of job? From a naturopathic perspective, when the stress of the situation is resolved, the blood pressure might return to normal, especially if the aggravating or contributing factors were also addressed. It is important for the patient to recognize how their body responded and to understand why. For example, if the patient was aware that the rise in blood pressure was due to how they handled the stressful situation, a more appropriate treatment strategy might be for the patient to learn new coping strategies. It is important for patients to continue to have their blood pressure monitored, but it might not be needed, or desirable, for them to continually take medication for a condition that they have resolved, especially if in the process they have learned new coping strategies. If, on the other hand, the blood pressure does not return to normal, a naturopathic doctor would look for other aggravating factors, such as diet or lifestyle and would assess if the situation was completely resolved, i.e. is the patient still angry about the separation, do they still fear that they will lose their job again, are they apprehensive about getting into another relationship, did they settle for a job with less pay or status?

Not all disease states can be resolved completely, but I would contend that there are many more than the current medical system acknowledges. The mind, that is a patient's intentions, beliefs and expectations, dictates the degree of change that is possible. I expect that practitioners of the future will spend more time with patients addressing the limitations that they impose on themselves. Making the unconscious conscious, and modifying intentions and beliefs can be done many ways, such as mindfulness exercises, meditation, yoga, journaling, 'talk therapy', etc. Also, changing language changes experiences and the impact of those experiences on health. Learning to reframe situations and to re-write the internal mental map is a valuable treatment strategy.

Verbal linking

When patients are conveying information to a practitioner they do so in a specific sequence. They link events and symptoms often unconsciously. This linking and sequencing of language is an important piece of the puzzle. It provides a guide to the factors that have contributed to the state of overwhelm and it indicates the factors that need to shift in order for healing to begin. For example, when a patient says, 'Ever since university I have had digestive problems', the practitioner then ask further questions to determine what changed in university, was it because of late nights, changes in dietary habits, increase in alcohol, stress because of grades, relationship issues, or something else.

Energy of words

For some people there is an upside to illness or disease. There is some benefit or result that they desire. For example, a patient who is in a car accident and finds that since the accident her family is helping out more around the house. If the patient is concerned that when she gets well she will have to go back to doing most of the work on her own she may consciously, or unconsciously, block the healing process. Addressing the impact of any disease or injury, both the positives and negatives, provides a practitioner, and often a patient, with insight into any factors that might be contributing to the healing process being inhibited.

The impact of words is especially relevant when it comes to the labeling of diseases and the conveying of the relationship between symptoms, disease, and a patient's life. Words have energy, and there are symbolic meanings to many diseases that have an impact on a patient's perception of their ability to heal (Benor 2006). For example, the fear associated with the diagnosis of cancer, the chronic debility associated with arthritis, the anticipation of ongoing pain associated with the diagnosis of fibromyalgia. Words either create boundaries or opportunities. The words that a patient associates with their symptoms and disease convey not only the nature and characteristics of the symptoms, but the symbolic meaning.

A patient's language reveals a contracted or supportive state. When the body is contracted, healing and health are restricted. In a supportive state, a patient has more choice, more movement, and more 'space'. By bringing a patient's awareness to their language, and assisting them in reframing it, you can stimulate the healing process. The following is a list of contracted language:

- 'not good enough'
- 'have no control'
- 'not safe'
- 'stuck'
- 'not strong enough'
- 'no support'

The following is a list of supportive language:

- 'secure'
- 'grateful'
- 'confident'
- 'doing well'

- 'relaxed'
- 'enthusiastic'
- 'loved'
- 'supported'
- 'strong'

Speech patterns

Speed, volume, tone, pitch, and texture of a voice all display an energetic pattern. As a patient speaks of events or people that affect them, one or more of the speech patterns will change. The specific change relates to the impact of that event and the uniqueness of each patient. Assessing speech patterns requires developing your listening skills, really listening to the details in someone's speech, and evaluating the relationship that a patient's voice has to their energetic patterns. What you are listening for is the congruence between what a patient is talking about and how they say it. Sometimes you hear the presence of an elemental quality. For example, a patient's speech is slow and monotonous as they tell you the details of a story, indicating the presence of earth. Other times what stands out is the lack of an element. For example, someone who looks very fiery (fit, red complexion, muscular build) and is talking about an event that they say was very exciting, but their voice is slow, and has a low monotone pitch (an earth quality). The absence of fire is as relevant as the presence of earth. When listening to a conversation, look for both. Are the elements present or absent, strong or weak? Listening to a patient's speech involves interest not just in what the participant says, but also in silences, in the rate and pitch of how they speak, in breathing, and so on. It is about paying attention to all aspects and recognizing that they are all important.

'The spoken language is the most important diagnostic and therapeutic tool in medicine' (The Editors 2001). It conveys much more than most practitioners or patients recognize as voice changes in response to internal and external stimuli and it mirrors the energetic shifts in the body. Voice displays an elemental quality in the following ways.

- An *earth* pattern is deep, resonant, and monotonous. It is low in pitch and slow. The conversation has specific points and a structure. There is a definite start and end to the conversation. When you are talking with a patient who has earth qualities there is a tendency for their answers to be either really short and to the point or to be really detailed. Earth patients are better with dates and times. They tend to be more comfortable with questions that are structured, that ask for something specific. When they are telling you about a health concern it contains a lot of facts, in a logical sequence. The following is an example of an earth patient recalling an accident: 'On Friday, May 15 at 3:40 p.m. I was turning right onto O'Connor Street and a green Ford ran the red light and hit the rear fender of my new Chevrolet Impala that I just bought on April 3. My car spun ½ way around and my left eyebrow hit the steering wheel. I had a constant, throbbing headache over my left eye for 3 ½ days. Since then I get a headache every 3 to 4 days. The headache lasts for about 2 hours. It is better if I lie down or if I drink something warm.

- A *water* pattern flows and is gentle. It has more of a connected story characteristic. Water answers tend to be long winded, yet not necessarily full of a lot of details. You might ask a question about one thing and the patient answering adds so many other extraneous details that the point is lost. If a water patient was telling about the car accident above it would sound more like this, 'May was a busy month. My sister wasn't feeling very well and work was really busy because we had this new project we were doing. I was leaving work early one Friday to go and see my sister and I was in a car accident. The lady that hit me was really upset, but she was okay. There were a number of people who came to see if I was all right. My eye and my head hurt for a while after the accident. Since then I get headaches more often.

- *Fire* has more flare, volume, and direction. The voice is sharp and short with a staccato timbre. A conversation with a fire patient tends to have more extremes of emotion with a focus and intensity on a few points. Aspects of the story leap out at you. If a patient with a lot of fire qualities was talking about the car accident it would sound more like this: 'In May, this crazy women ran a red light and hit my new car. The pain in my eye was excruciating. For days it felt like there was a hammer inside my head. Months later I'm still having these stupid headaches. I just want to know what I can do to fix these headaches.

- An *air* voice is breathy with quick changes in context. It comes across as disjointed and often with a higher pitch. Patients with air qualities have a greater tendency to convey facts more randomly without a lot of details. It is more about the impression that events have had on them and how that triggered other events. If an air patient was talking about the car accident it would sound more like this, 'I have these headaches that sometimes bother me. My arm bothers me too. It was hurt when I fell off my bike not in the car accident.

- The quality of *ether* is conveyed in a patient's freedom of expression. When ether is lacking, an obvious restriction is heard. The voice is squeaky without flexibility or range in pitch, volume, rate, or tone. When ether is present the true quality of the patient comes through. The voice is open. Expression is easy and unguarded.

- A patient who is *internally focused* would emphasize the symptoms as a result of the accident, such as, 'The headache is so bad that it disrupts my sleep. It also affects my ability to work out as much as working out aggravates my headaches and they are also affecting my energy and my mood.'

- A patient who is *externally focused* would emphasize how the accident affects their ability to fulfill their responsibilities to others, such as, 'Ever since the accident I am not able to do as much around the house, my husband has to take on more of the responsibilities, and he is already really busy at work. Also, I am not able to concentrate as much at work which is impacting my job and others are relying on me, I hate letting them down.'

Listening

Listening involves letting patients speak without interrupting, without dictating the order of the information, and the way that it is conveyed. Listening is a valuable skill that takes practice, patience, and intention. Many factors interfere with listening, such as a practitioner's desire to help, their anxieties, something in the patient's story might trigger an unresolved issue in the practitioner, or the practitioner might be feeling sleepy, angry, hateful, pre-occupied, etc. (Proner 2006).

Patients want their doctors to listen to them, to understand their concerns, to help them understand what is happening to their bodies, to reassure them, and to help them heal (Platt & Gordon 2004). An important skill for a practitioner is that of listening and paying attention to all that a patient is conveying.

> *This attention to detail – the importance of taking seriously all that the patient has to say about the illness, and the belief that it all matters and has meaning – is a healing process in itself. It encourages the patient to see themselves as an integrated whole (Swayne 1998).*

Listening to patients is both a receptive and an active process. A practitioner knows what they need to undercover in the intake, but the therapeutic value of the intake is to allow the patient to express, especially initially, in the way that is natural for them. The practitioner's role is to listen for key words and phrases, and to develop an understanding of what the patient is conveying consciously and unconsciously. Initially, the role of the practitioner is to be receptive to what and how the patient chooses to express themself. The process becomes active as the practitioner attempts to put all the pieces together, by asking pertinent questions and then listening to the patient's answers in order to complete the puzzle.

Remember that symptoms and diseases are not just relevant to patients because they alter physiological functions in the body; they are relevant because they alter a patient's life. 'Listen to your patient.' Find out how they are experiencing their illness, what impact it has had on their life, and on their sense of self. What are their fears, concerns, thoughts, and desires? It is by listening that we include the human element into the understanding of health and disease.

Non-verbal behavior

Patients are able to consciously control what they will or won't say, but the reactions of the body in response to emotions, thoughts, and language are primarily unconscious and hence often can convey as much or more than a patient's actual words.

> *Since nonverbal behavior is under less conscious control than words, when there is a lack of congruence between the two, the nonverbal message is likely to be more representative of the patient's real attitudes and feelings (Bernstein & Bernstein 1985).*

Posture, gestures, blushing, a frown, a smile, a change in tone of voice all convey relevant information.

> *The postural language of the body, the bodily expression of emotions, and the total pre-verbal behavior, such as symptomatic actions, are generally interpreted in terms of unconscious motivation (Thass-Thienemann 1968).*

The therapeutic encounter

There are many books written on the meanings of various non-verbal behaviors. Caution must be encouraged when interpreting a patient's behavior. A frown, for example, might indicate annoyance, it might indicate concentration, or it might just be a habit for a patient. Folding of one's arms might be a sign of being closed off, it might indicate a comfortable position due to pain or injury, or it might simply indicate the patient is feeling cold. From an assessment point of view, I encourage you to pay attention to the energetics of the non-verbal behavior and to recognize the generalities of the concepts, for example:

- *Air* movements tend to wander around the body; they appear first in one arm, then a leg, then somewhere else. They tend to affect the nervous system and breathing, such as a twitching eye or periodic jerking of the arm or leg.
- *Fire* behavior has a direction, a force and intensity to it. It usually relates to single part or spot on the body that has varying degrees of restlessness, irritability, redness, or heat.
- *Water* movement naturally is flowing. It has a sway or an embracing precise, definitive quality. When in a state of disharmony, it may manifest as a lack of flow, or a build up fluid that impedes the flow.
- *Earth* behavior is slow, steady, consistent, plodding in nature, and heavy or stiff.

Non-verbal behavior is conveyed by the patient to the practitioner and by the practitioner to the patient. Looking at your watch, or becoming restless or distracted, all convey impatience or a lack of interest in the patient. The eye contact of the practitioner, the distance between the patient and the practitioner, the disparity in height of chairs, or the angle of chairs also convey meaning to a patient. For example, 'Patients tend to feel greater anxiety when the interviewer is positioned more than about three feet from the patient. Obviously, extreme proximity can also frighten the patient' (Bernstein & Bersntein 1985). Just as a practitioner uses the patient's non-verbal behavior to indicate the significance of something, a patient will likely confer meaning to practitioner's non-verbal behavior.

Changes in affect

When a memory, event, situation, or person brings up emotion when it is being talked about, it is affecting health; either positively or negatively. For example, when a patient is talking about the new love of their life, or their recent promotion, or the pride of graduating you expect to hear an increase in the liveliness and energy of voice. If someone is talking about an abusive situation or a traumatic incident that still affects them you would hear a drop in the tone, speed, and a shift in the energetic quality of their voice.

Every situation that affects a patient carries a charge, that is, it triggers them on some level. The degree and type of charge reflects the degree and type of impact. When a patient talks about something that affects them, there is a change in their affect, that is, in their verbal or non-verbal behavior. If you listen to a patient's voice as a wave pattern what you notice is a change in the qualities of the wave; for example, a patient might start off talking

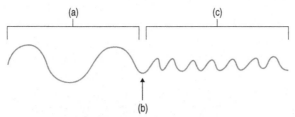

Fig 8.2 Changes in affect (a) Normal voice pattern; (b) trigger (mention of a situation or event that is unresolved for a patient); (c) voice pattern when triggered.

about their family with a certain tone. As soon as they mention a specific person there is change in the tone, that is, it might drop or rise, the rate of speech increases or decreases, or there is an overt display of emotion, or an obvious guarding of emotion. Something in the way they talk changes in response to that person or event (see Fig 8.2).

When you hear a change in affect, explore it further. Ask the patient to expand on what they were saying. Ask about the person or situation. Find out how much of an impact this person, event, or situation holds. Look for the correlation between the charged event and the onset of any of the patient's symptoms. The concept 'the layers of life' is a symbolic representation of how situations and events affect a patient's state of health (refer to Chapter 5).

Changes in affect relate to the interaction of language and emotion, both consciously and unconsciously. When a patient is actively involved in a current situation, it is healthy to show emotion. When the expression of emotion is in alignment and in coherence with how a patient feels about the situation, the more likely the act of expressing assists in resolving the situation. For example, if a patient is frustrated with a situation at work and they express their frustration, either at the time or later, they are more likely to feel better. When a patient recalls a situation from their past and the situation still 'triggers' them there is a very strong chance that the impact of the situation was never completely resolved and that it is still impacting their health.

Often the degree of affect change is an indicator of the degree of its importance. For example, when a patient is recalling a motor vehicle accident that happened 3 years ago and you can see by their body posture that they are still 'triggered' and as they tell their story it sounds as if the accident happened yesterday. This would indicate that the body is still in the state of overwhelm due to the accident. Having patients explore situations that cause a change in affect, through free-form writing, journaling, art exercises, referral to a psychologist, or other means, might be an effective way of having them understand the impact that the situations have had on their life. Awareness and intention is important to assist a patient in 'unwinding' and resolving the emotional charges of past events and situations.

Somatic metaphors

A somatic metaphor (Fig. 8.3) is when a physical disease appears to be 'saying' the same thing, expressing the same meaning, as the patient's subjective 'story' conveyed in verbal language (Broom 2002). Symptoms imply meaning and they can convey what a patient is unable to express or what they are unable to adequately process. There often is a close mirroring

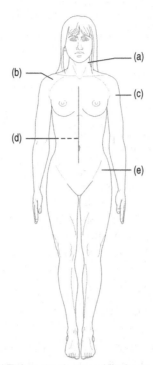

Fig 8.3 Somatic metaphors. (a) Tightness in throat or difficulty swallowing – does not feel that they can speak up or say what they really want to say. (b) Tightness in shoulders – feeling like they are carrying the weight of the world – too many responsibilities. (c) Decrease in range of motion of shoulder – not taking what they need from life or not letting go of what they do not need. (d) Weakness in back – not feeling supported or strong. (e) Pain and stiffness in hips – a feeling of being restricted and not being able to move forward in life.

between a patient's words and phrases, what they say, think, and feel, and what is happening on a functional and structural level. 'In all languages there are words and concepts with dual meanings relating to both sensor-motor and mental systems' (Mattsson & Mattsson 2002).

Their words indicate what the energy is doing. A patient often describes their symptoms using the same terminology to describe their life. For example, a patient who feels that they are being constricted by their life often feels constriction in their body. A patient who feels frustrated, often has a condition, such as a skin rash, that is itchy and frustrating to them. When asking clarifying questions, it is helpful to stay in the patient's language and to ask questions using the words that a patient has used. For example, if a patient says that they feel a lot of heaviness in their legs and it is difficult to move you might ask them if there is any situation in their life that seems heavy and isn't shifting or moving.

Examples of key words and phrases are:

- 'It feels like there is a weight on my shoulders.'
- 'There is a lot of pressure on my chest.'
- 'I don't have enough time.'
- 'I feel stuck.'
- 'My knee just doesn't want to move forward.'

- 'I don't feel supported.'
- 'I feel restricted.'
- 'I feel weak.'

When a patient uses these key words and phrases, pay attention to how the symbolism of their words mirrors their health concerns, and then ask them a broad follow up question. For example, from the previous key words and phrases, a practitioner might ask:

- 'What does the weight on your shoulders represent?'
- 'Tell me about the pressure on your chest? Is there any part of your life that feels pressured?'
- 'Not enough time to do what? What would you like to do if you have more time?'
- 'Tell me about feeling stuck. Is there anywhere else in your life where you feel stuck?'
- 'Tell me about moving forward in your life.'
- 'In what way do you not feel supported in your life.'
- 'Tell me more about feeling restricted.'
- 'Where do you feel weakness in your body?'

By following up on key words and phrases a practitioner is able to delve deeper into the root causes of the energetic shifts. Most patients understand that there is a link between their life and their health; what they don't understand is the degree. When the correlation between symptoms and situations is brought to a patient's awareness it provides them with immediate feedback on how their body responds; and hence with more options of how they can influence their life and their health. When looking at the linkage between a patient's symptoms and their life, it is important to remember that diseases, although logical, are multi-factorial. It is important not to 'blame' a patient. The value of somatic metaphors is that they provide a guide, or a clue, as to what needs to change in order to restore health.

The symbolic meaning of illness and disease is ingrained in the medical profession; but often unrecognized and unacknowledged. For example, it is common for a practitioner to advise a patient with hypertension to 'take it easy, to relax more' or to advise a patient with anxiety to 'slow down and not worry as much'. This implies that, on some level, the practitioner is aware that a psychological state has triggered or contributed to the manifestation of physiological symptoms. Being able to link the two, in a way that makes sense to a patient, is of more value than an 'off the cuff' remark that has no frame of reference.

QUESTIONING

During an assessment, the practitioner's role is to ask the questions that reveal the initiating, aggravating, and ameliorating factors. Questions also are helpful in understanding the full nature of symptoms and the depth of their impact on health. Generally, the practitioner talks as little as possible, especially at the start of the initial intake, and allows the patient to do the majority of the talking, uninterrupted.

The style and type of questions used depends on the age and health status of the patient. There are many factors that need to be taken into consideration; including, language barriers, speech and hearing difficulties, dementia and organic brain syndromes, current health status of the patient, and their level of discomfort and pain. The purpose of this book is limited to the energetics of questions and how they reveal the underlying root cause and aggravating factors.

Start with open-ended questions

Open-ended questions can *not* be answered with a 'yes' or 'no'. They have a broad focus and allow the patient to tell their story in the way they have it stored. 'Skill at asking such questions probably determines one's success as a physician more than any other factor' (Orient 2005). Initially, open-ended questions convey whether a patient has an internal or an external focus. They allow the practitioner to see how a patient connects their health to their life. The broader the open-ended question, the more information you gather.

Some patients are uncomfortable with broad questions, yet I encourage you to ask a very open-ended question the first time you meet someone. For example, 'Tell me about yourself'. This allows patients the greatest opportunity to display their true energetic qualities. If this type of questioning is too broad for a patient, they will ask a clarifying question or they will narrow the scope with what they tell you. In follow-up visits, start with an open-ended question, such as 'What brings you in today?' or 'How have you been?' Questions such as 'tell me about your pain,' or 'is your digestion better?' lead the patient to focus on a specific aspect of their health and you often miss changes in the overall pattern, or the onset of new signs and symptoms due to recent changes or events in a patient's life.

Continue with open-ended questions

After the patient has responded to your first open-ended question, ask questions that follow up on key words and phrases that they have used, that is, stay in the language of the patient. The more you mirror the language of the patient, the more comfortable they will feel. The main exception is when a patient uses profanity or jargon. The goal is for the practitioner and patient to see the connections, to understand the impact between what has happened, and what is going on with the body.

> *The physician obtains more precise information respecting each particular detail, but without ever framing his questions so as to suggest the answer to the patients (Hahnemann 1996).*

Ask clarifying questions

Only after a patient has had the opportunity to respond to open ended questions do you ask clarifying questions. These questions are useful to ensure that the patient and the practitioner are speaking the same language.

Practitioners need to be careful not to use medical jargon and they need to recognize that a patient's description of body parts is not always as it seems. For example,

> The use of the patient's own words might preclude a precise description at that point. The pain in the 'tummy' might be in the epigastrium, hypochondrium, periumbilical area, suprapubic area or even the colon and rectum (Orient 2005).

Use simple, clear words. Stay in the language of the patient, as much as possible. When there is any doubt as to the precise meaning of a patient's words, especially as they relate to parts of the body, ask the patient to demonstrate and point to the part of the body they are talking about.

Clarifying questions shed light on the nature of the symptoms and the status of key indicators to health. Each symptom and each clinical system has its own specific clarifying questions that are relevant. For example, if the symptom involved the respiratory system, you would ask clarifying questions with respect to cough, sputum production, hemoptysis, chest pain, shortness of breath, wheezing, etc. You would also ask questions about smoking, time spent inside versus outside, impact of exertion on breathing, the use of chemicals and sprays at home and work, the type of cleaning products, and the impact of environment on symptoms, etc. If the symptom was pain, you would ask clarifying questions about the site of the pain, the characteristics, onset, progression, duration, intensity, frequency, depth if it radiates, and other symptoms that are associated with it, as well as what aggravates or alleviates it.

Clarifying questions include the characteristics of the symptoms, and the relevant lifestyle factors, environmental and external factors. They also include detailed questions about the building blocks to health. The following are examples of the questions that might be asked for some of the building blocks to health.

Food

- type of food a patient eats
- the quantity and proportions of different types of food
- how they prepare and cook their food
- their eating regimen and the environment that they eat in
- what they drink when they are eating and how much they drink
- who they eat with and what they do when they are eating
- their food intolerances and their likes and dislikes
- their beliefs about food and eating.

Every aspect of what a patient conveys has meaning and is relevant. For many patients, the most valuable piece of advice that a practitioner can provide is simple change that has a profound effect on health, such as not drinking water when you eat, especially if a patient has hypochlorhydria; or eating smaller, more frequent meals, if a patient has hypoglycemia; or explaining to a patient that their digestion is likely to be better simply by relaxing when they eat and allowing the body to digest their food.

Sleep

- their consumption of caffeine – when and how much
- their consumption of sugar, chocolate, fruit and other food that is known to disrupt sleep
- their eating patterns, how late their last meal is and whether they snack before bed
- their mental activity, their concerns and worries and how they handle them
- their level of activity or inactivity
- the amount of time that they spend outside in a day and the presence of fluorescent lights in their home and work environment
- the type of job they have and whether it involves shift work or long hours
- the type of house and neighborhood they live in and how many people live in the house
- the amount of time they spend in front of the television or on the computer
- what activities they do in the bedroom, such as reading and watching television
- their bedroom regimen
- the amount of darkness and noise they hear when trying to sleep
- what wakes them up at night – noise, young children, need to use the bathroom, pain or discomfort, their mind chatter, etc.
- whether they have a problem falling asleep, whether they wake often, wake early or they just wake up after a night's sleep still feeling tired.

Insomnia, or problems with sleeping, is a very common symptom. Addressing the underlying cause depends on understanding the factors that contribute to the problem. With some patients that I have treated the recommendations have been as simple as changing their curtains so the streetlights don't shine into their bedroom; others have found that by stopping eating 3 hours before bed, or eliminating caffeine and sugar earlier in the day was the answer; for others it involves addressing internal mind chatter and worry. Knowing the particulars about sleeping patterns is important. The solution might be very simple, or the pattern of sleeping concerns might indicate a much deeper problem that needs to be addressed, such as blood deficiency syndrome, cirrhosis, heart problems, respiratory problems, hyperthyroidism, etc. (Collins 1997).

Lifestyle energy

A patient's lifestyle has an energetic pattern that consequently impacts their health. Lifestyle questions inquire about a patient's daily regimen, job, hobbies, etc. Find out what they do and what they think of what they do. Do they love the hurriedness and excitement of their day, or does it cause them constant stress and discomfort? The following is an overview of how to look at lifestyle elementally.

- An *internally* focused lifestyle involves a patient doing a lot for themselves. They take time to ensure that they are eating correctly, exercising enough, getting enough sleep and relaxing and enjoying life. They pay attention to the signs and symptoms that indicate disharmony in their body. They take responsibility for ensuring that they live a healthy lifestyle.

- An *externally* focused lifestyle involves paying attention to the duties and responsibilities that one has for other people. Personal factors, such as eating, drinking water, sleeping, and exercise are put on hold as 'there isn't enough time' or there are other people or external projects that take priority.
- *Earth* lifestyle is structured, routine, and consistent. Too much *earth* results in feeling bored, closed in, or stuck; too little causes feelings of insecurity, or a sense that not enough is being accomplished.
- *Water* lifestyle flows. It revolves around relationships with people or things. An imbalanced water lifestyle involves taking care of others to excess and not taking care or nurturing yourself, or the other way around. It involves taking on more and more all the time, like a flowing river that picks up everything in its path.
- A *fire* lifestyle is busy and active. When there is a fire imbalance, a patient complains of not having enough time, not being able to do things fast enough, or not being able to focus. A lack of fire shows up when someone finds they lack passion, enthusiasm, direction, or motivation.
- An *air* lifestyle changes constantly and quickly. There is diversity and spontaneity. Many tasks are started and few are ever finished. Too much air shows up as feeling scattered and unable to complete any task; too little shows up as being stifled, stale or impatient because of the lack of variety in life.
- The *ether* aspect shows up in a patient's will to live and in the enjoyment they find in their life. There is an overall sense of energy and enjoyment in life.

Ask awareness questions

Awareness questions are questions that provide further details on the nature of symptoms and assist a patient in seeing the link between their health concerns and their life. For example: If you think of that situation right now, what do you notice in your body? What was going on in your life when the symptoms started? The last time you had stomach pains do you remember what you were doing at that time?

When asking awareness questions avoid leading the patient. Patients might agree with a practitioner simply to avoid exploring a point in more detail, or because they don't want to admit that they don't know. It is helpful to provide a patient with multiple options. This provides them with the knowledge that there is not just one answer, and it provides them with information that can increase their awareness in the future. For example, if a patient complains of gas, instead of asking if it is worse after eating a meal you might ask, 'When is the gas the worst, first thing in the morning, just after eating, about two hours about eating, or is it worse as the day goes on? Is the gas constant, weekly or periodically?' Patients initially are unaware of a lot of the details of their symptoms. Part of the intake, and part of the process of working to improve health, is to provide patients with a concept of what is normal versus common, what different symptoms relate to, and the importance of being more aware of their reaction to different aspects of their life. The more that patients have a framework for health and disease and the more they are aware of and look for correlations between their symptoms and their lifestyle, the more options they have to maintain a higher level of health. Sometimes the awareness questions are given as 'homework' to encourage patients to have a better understanding of the nature of their symptoms, what aggravates and what ameliorates them.

When patients are overwhelmed with their symptoms and report that they have 'always' been tired, or in pain, or had insomnia, or whatever the symptom is, a good question is, 'When is the last time you can remember feeling perfectly healthy?' Having a patient focus on the time periods of their life when they were symptom free often provides a better indicator as to what factors have impacted their health. With some symptoms, such as pain, patients can be focused on the pain and it can override their awareness of parts of the body that are pain free. When a patient reports that the 'everything' hurts, it is helpful to have a patient focus on and identify parts of the body that aren't in pain, such as their toes, or their abdomen.

Ask compliance questions

Working holistically, often involves a patient making changes in their lifestyle. It involves dietary changes, ensuring sufficient water intake, and ensuring that exercise and sleep are a regular part of their daily regimen. Living a life that is conducive to health is essential if you expect to be healthy. In follow-up visits with patients, it is important to ask about their compliance with the changes and treatment plans that were prescribed. Asking a patient about their compliance to 'their homework' is best done prior to inquiring about their change in symptoms. It is better to ask a question such as, 'Are you finding it easy to follow the dietary program?' instead of 'Are you following the dietary program?' The first example has less implied judgment and is more likely to get a patient to open up about the aspects that they found difficult.

A patient makes changes so that they achieve the health goals that they have set, they don't make changes for their practitioner. It is important that a practitioner keep the focus of treatment on what the patient does. It is the patient that heals themself, it is not the practitioner that does the healing. If a patient is concerned with pleasing a practitioner, or hesitant that they have disappointed their practitioner, then the emphasis of the treatment is on the practitioner, and needs to be changed so that the patient recognizes and owns the treatment plan. Their motivation needs to be their health; not the opinion of their practitioner.

Stay focused on the pattern

By the nature of the questioning, during a holistic intake, a patient reveals more information than is typical in a conventional medical history taking. It is important that a practitioner focus on the patterns that are emerging throughout the questioning process and that they stay out of the details of the story. For example, if a patient is talking about an argument with their spouse what is relevant is the impact that the argument had on the patient and why; not the details of the argument. It is about hearing the connection between life events and situations that aggravate symptoms; what isn't important is what someone said next, or what happened next in a story. A practitioner's job is to ensure that the therapeutic encounter is therapeutic, not merely conversational. What is important is how an event or situation has impacted a patient, not the details of the event. There is a very distinct difference between a detailed therapeutic holistic intake, and a chat with a good friend.

WILLINGNESS TO HEAL

Throughout the holistic intake a patient reveals their willingness to heal through the words they choose and how they talk about their health. As patients talk their internal mind chatter is revealed. What you are listening for is whether they spend time focused on healing or being sick. Do they see the world as positive or negative? Is there a negative event that they can't seem to let go of? What associations do they make with respect to their state of health? You are listening for whether their mind is helping them heal or contributing to disease. Research shows that the more a patient believes something will help them, the more it does. Likewise, you can provide the body with the right treatment, but if their mind is reinforcing a disease state, the treatment will be less effective or not effective at all (Fosha 2006, Chow & Tsang 2007).

Disease and illness, for some, serves a purpose, it allows a patient to do or not do something. For example, a patient finds that after an accident her family members help out around the house a lot more. In a way, the symptoms are a means of gaining control and expressing her anger. If the patient links getting well with having to do everything on her own again, it might inhibit the healing process. Another example is a patient was diagnosed with fibromyalgia who enjoyed the support and attention that she received from the support group. As a result, she was unwilling, on an unconscious level, to get well as she would lose 'her new friends'. For example, when you ask a patient what will happen when they are pain free and their initial response is to 'fight that idea', such as saying 'I would like the pain to decrease, but I don't expect it to ever go completely away', there is a strong indicator that the pain is serving an underlying purpose and this purpose needs to be addressed in order for a patient, on a conscious and unconscious level, to allow the body to heal.

QUESTIONNAIRES

There is a lot of essential information that needs to be gathered during a visit, especially the initial visit. Questionnaires are an efficient way to gather this information. I find that questionnaires, especially if they are lengthy, are the most helpful when they are sent to a patient prior to the initial visit. This provides them time to gather all the relevant information, to verify dates, and increase their awareness of their health; not only for their chief concerns but on all aspects. Questionnaires provide a framework for the breadth and depth of questioning that will be asked during the initial visit and assists in

The therapeutic encounter

preparing a patient for the visit. A questionnaire needs to reflect the practitioner in style and breadth of questions. It often is the first introduction that a patient has to a practitioner. If a questionnaire is really short and to the point and then the practitioner asks questions that are more personal and probing, a patient is likely to feel more guarded. If, on the other hand, a questionnaire is very extensive and involves the patient conveying a lot of personal information, that is disregarded or not followed up on during the session, it too affects the patient's comfort level with the practitioner.

Questionnaires are helpful to fill in the blanks for items that don't come up during the initial conversation, to provide details for a wide range of health concerns, and to cover family history, medications and supplements, allergies, major life events, and history of accidents, injuries, surgeons, and medical procedures. Questionnaires also provide insight into a patient's ability to recall past events. The presence or absence of detail and how they list health concerns provides information on their elemental quality. For example, a patient with earth qualities provides a lot of detail, with precise dates, and in a chronological order; a patient with fire qualities tends to focus on a specific symptom.

Listen to what a patient thinks of the questionnaire: do they find it too long, too detailed, and/or too personal? It is all relevant and part of the energetic picture. Also, the questions that are omitted by the patient provide a heads-up for the practitioner as to what the patient might not be open to discussing or aspects of their life they can't recall. For example, if a questionnaire asks about past abuse or addictions and the patient answers this section, there is a greater likelihood that they will be prepared to discuss those issues. If, on the other hand, a patient leaves them blank it might indicate that these topics are not as easy for them to discuss. It doesn't mean that as a practitioner you don't address these questions, it just provides you information as to the comfort level of the patient.

Questionnaires can be used throughout the course of working with a patient. At any time a questionnaire is a valuable tool to expand on an area of concern, to assist a patient and the practitioner in deepening the awareness and understanding of an energetic pattern, and in tracking the progress and change in key symptoms, such as pain or range of motion. It is also valuable to repeat aspects of the questionnaire, such as the review of systems, throughout a treatment process or on a yearly basis, as a way of tracking progress and seeing how the patterns change and the improvement in health, or the progression of disease.

At the start of the intake allow the patient to speak freely and avoid starting with the questionnaire. An undirected initial focus provides a strong indication for the aspects of their life that are the most involved in their health and their disease. The value of a questionnaire is that it 'fills in the blanks' for the other aspects of health, ensuring that a practitioner has as many pieces of the puzzle as possible and ensuring that key information is not omitted.

A holistic medical questionnaire includes the following information:

- *Family history*. A patient's family history relates major illnesses or disease that parents, grandparents, and siblings have incurred. It relates to their marital status and the presence of children. It includes an overview of the support network that their family provides, how close the family is, and the responsibilities associated with their family. During the family history, a practitioner gets an idea of the degree to which immediate family and extended family impact the health of the patient. For example, sick children, aging parents, and dysfunctional family dynamics can all be major stressors for a patient. On the other hand, loving parents, strong family network, and closeness of siblings can provide a lot of support and can assist in off-setting the stress of other factors.

- *Medical history.* Medical history involves a chronological listing of all accidents, injuries, surgeries, illness, and major health events in a patient's life. It includes clarification on the type of treatments that were used, both conventional and complementary, the healing process and the outcomes. It involves a listing of all past and current medications – both prescription and over-the-counter, all supplements including herbal remedies, homeopathics, and nutraceuticals. It is important to note all allergies and adverse or questionable reactions to drugs or supplements. A medical history also involves the listing of all medical procedures, cosmetic or reconstructive surgeries, dental work, special diets, or health programs that a patient has engaged in. A complete review of systems needs to be included as well as a listing of all past and current health concerns. The purpose of a detailed medical history is for the practitioner to have a sense of the timing and progression of symptoms. To see the relationship between major events and the onset of symptoms, and to recognize any key factors that might be contributing to the current symptoms or disease state.
- *Lifestyle.* Reviewing a patient's lifestyle and daily regimen provides a practitioner with an idea of the patient's awareness of what a healthy lifestyle is and to what degree they are following it. By reviewing all aspects of the building blocks to health, a practitioner will have an idea of which ones might be contributing to a patient's symptoms, and for how long they have been imbalanced.
- *Social and environmental history.* Asking questions about a patient's alcohol and smoking habits, whether they have a history of drug use, as well as their sexual history. Knowing a patient's hobbies, how often they take a vacation, and where they travel is also important. For example, where a patient vacations provides insight to the exposure to pathogens, information as to whether a patient prefers solitude or excitement, nature or cities. The review also includes the type of house that they grew up in and that they currently live in, how the house is heated, the water source, etc. It also includes a patient's employment history with a focus on the type of materials that they have had exposure to and the amount of stress or impact their job has had on their life. Where a patient was born and any industries and manufacturing that were in close proximity are also important. The aim of the social and environmental questioning is to identify any relevant factors. For example, a patient might be currently living in Toronto, but grew up in Nova Scotia. If their chief complaint is melanoma that point is relevant as many parts of Nova Scotia have high levels of arsenic in the soil and there is a known correlation between high

arsenic levels and skin cancer (Walvekar et al 2007). It is not the patient's job to be aware of the significance of the factors; it is the role of the practitioner.

- *Mental state.* Throughout the history taking a patient conveys their mental state: their thoughts and feelings about their disease, their health goals, and their expectations. The mental state of the assessment is a critical aspect of the process as it sets the direction, determines the likelihood of the journey being successful, and provides a practitioner with an idea of whether or not all aspects of a patient are willing and able to make the necessary changes.

RECORD KEEPING

Record keeping is an integral part of the interviewing process. There are legal and moral responsibilities for maintaining accurate records of all patient contacts. In addition, accurate records allow a practitioner to refresh their memory about the details of previous sessions, the treatment strategy, the changes in lifestyle or behavior that they are monitoring, and to assess progress.

It is important to retain the language of the patient in the record keeping. When a practitioner is looking for the patterns between a patient's story and their symptoms, it is important that the words and phrases of the patient be captured.

ASSESSMENT OUTCOMES

The assessment process is the most important part of the therapeutic encounter. Everything else, the diagnosis and the treatment, depend on a thorough and accurate assessment. Every patient is an individual and treatments are individually based on the uniqueness of the patient. The more fully a practitioner understands their patient, the more likely they will determine not only a treatment plan, but a communication plan that works for each patient. A stronger patient–practitioner relationship, coupled with a thorough assessment, provides a practitioner with the required pieces to accurately diagnose not only what is going on with a patient, but why.

The following assessment outcomes require information from the holistic intake and from the physical assessment. These outcomes guide a practitioner in their diagnosis and in determining a treatment strategy for each patient.

- patient's constitution
- current level of vitality
- level of the shift
- symptom patterns
- initiating factors
- aggravating factors
- risk to health
- patient's beliefs and expectations
- patient's healing intention
- resources for healing and change.

Assessment is the process of observing, listening, analyzing, and collecting data from a patient; diagnosis is the identification or labeling of the findings from the assessment. People are assessed; symptoms and diseases are diagnosed. Each system of medicine has its own language and way of classifying symptoms and diseases. The way that diseases are classified greatly influences the treatment approach that is used. For example, traditional medical systems classify diseases according to their qualities and characteristics, such as excess Yang, deficient heat, liver congestion. These classifications guide the treatment strategy and the herbs, foods, or therapies used are chosen based on their ability to balance or harmonize the symptom and disease patterns.

Diagnoses provide a common language enabling medical professionals to correspond and to communicate. The vast knowledge that we have about anatomy, physiology, and pathology allows us to understand the workings of the human body in infinite detail. This knowledge has resulted in conventional diagnoses that are based on reductionist and dualistic concepts and hence have no link to the concept of human beings as complex interrelated systems that are affected by their environment. Conventional diagnoses might be a starting point, but they are not an efficient way of communicating the what, how, and why, of the disease to the patient. The diagnosing of disease is valuable when it takes into consideration what the disease means to the patient, the effect of their suffering and the way that their disease has impacted their life (Baron 1985). A diagnosis is valuable when it provides a patient with knowledge about how and what *they need to do* to restore wellness.

Many patients seek naturopathic medical care when there is no clear conventional diagnosis to explain their symptoms, or when they are in a chronic state or have multiple diagnoses. The focus of a naturopathic medical assessment is to identify the overriding pattern, the initiating and aggravating factors behind disease, to determine the progression of disease, and to determine the factors that need to be addressed in order to stimulate the inherent healing potential of the body. Hence, a naturopathic diagnosis might list the relevant conventional diagnoses, the clinical systems that are manifesting the disharmony, the initiating and aggravating factors, and the qualities of the symptoms.

The term 'naturopathic diagnosis' has various connotations and has resulted in many discussions in the naturopathic profession. A naturopathic diagnosis is often explanatory, versus categorical, and relates back to causative factors. Conventional medical diagnosis is categorical and relates to the pathological manifestation of the condition; not the cause. Naturopathic medicine utilizes conventional medical diagnosis as an understanding of the pathological condition for a patient, but as conventional diagnosis seldom relates to the causative factors, naturopathic medicine often has multiple diagnoses for a single patient. For example, the diagnoses for a patient might include irritable bowel syndrome, intolerance to wheat and sugar, imbalance in lifestyle factors (insufficient sleep, working long hours, lack of exercise), and frustration due to a situation at work. The treatment strategy would address the food intolerances and lifestyle factors, coping strategies to address the frustration; and the prescription of therapeutics if warranted based on the severity and chronicity of the symptoms. The importance of any diagnosis is that it accurately guides the treatment plan, for both the patient and the practitioner, to ensure optimal healing (Magner 1992).

A correct diagnosis can only be made with a complete assessment and a correct treatment strategy can only be done with a correct diagnosis.

REFERENCES

Bandler R, Grinder J 1979 Frogs into Princes, Neuro Linguistic Programming. Real People Press, Utah

Baron RJ 1985 An introduction to medical phenomenology: I can't hear you while I'm listening. Ann Intern Med 103:606–611

Barrier PA, Li JT, Jensen NM 2003 Two words to improve physician-patient communication: What else? Mayo Clin Proc 78:211–214

Benor DJ 2006 Wholistic Healing. The Healing Potential in a Word – part III. Positive Health, Portsmouth

Bernstein L, Bernstein RS 1985 Interviewing, a guide for health professionals, fourth edition. Appleton-Century Crofts, Connecticut

Broom B 2002 Somatic metaphor: a clinical phenomenon pointing to a new model of disease, personhood and physical reality. Adv Mind-Body Med 18(1):16–30

Chow YW, Tsang HW 2007 Biopsychosocial effects of Qigong as a mindful exercise for people with anxiety disorders: a speculative review. J Altern Complemen Med 13(8):831–839

Collins RD 1997 Differential Diagnosis in Primary Care, second edition. Lippincott, Philadelphia

Duffin J 2007 History of Medicine. University of Toronto Press, Toronto

Fosha D 2006 Quantum transformation in trauma and treatment: traversing the crisis of healing change. J Clin Psychol 62(5):569–583

Hahnemann S 1996 Organon of the Medical Art. Birdcage Books, Washington

Magner LN 1992 A History of Medicine. Marcel Dekker, New York

Mattsson B, Mattsson M 2002 The concept of 'psychosomatic' in general practice.

Reflections on body language and a tentative model for understanding. Scand J Prim Health Care 20(1):35–138

McTaggart L 2002 The Field, the Quest for the Secret Force of the Universe. HarperCollins Publishers, Great Britian

Murphy M 1993 The Future of the Body, Explorations into the Further Evolution of Human Nature. Jeremy P Tarcher, Los Angeles

Orient JM 2005 Sapira's Art and Science of Bedside Diagnosis 3rd edition. Lippincott Williams & Wilkins, Philadelphia

Platt FW, Gordon GF 2004 Field Guide to the Difficult Patient Interview, second edition. Lippincott Williams & Wilkins, Philadelphia

Proner BD 2006 A word about words. J Anal Psychol 51:423–435

Swayne J 1998 Homeopathic therapeutics: many dimensions – or meaningless diversity? In Vickers A (ed) 1998 Examining Complementary Medicine. Stanley Thornes, Cheltenham

Thass-Thienemann T 1968 Symbolic Behavior. Washington Square Press, New York

The Editors 2001 Medical Writings – 'Tell me about yourself': The patient-centered interview. Ann Intern Med 134(11):1080

Walvekar RR, Kane SV, Nadkarni MS, Bagwan IN, Chaukar DA, D'Cruz AK 2007 Chronic arsenic poisoning: a global health issue – a report of multiple primary cancers. J Cutan Pathol 34:203–206

Welsby PD 2002 Clinical History Taking and Examinations, second edition. Churchill Livingstone, Edinburgh

FURTHER READING

Barsky AF 1981 Hidden reasons some patients visit doctors. Ann Intern Med 94(1):492–490

Bayer-Fetzer Conference 2001 Essential elements of communication in medical

encounters: The Kalamazoo consensus statement. Academic Medicine 76(4)

Beckman HB, Frankel RM 1984 The effect of physician behavior on the collection of data. Annals of Internal Medicine 101:692–696

Beers MH, Berkow R 1999 The Merck Manual of Diagnosis and Therapy, seventeenth edition. Merck Research Laboratories, New Jersey

Bickley LS, Hoekelman RA 1999 Physical Examination and History Taking, seventh edition. Lippincott, Philadelphia

Bridges MR 2006 Activating the corrective emotional experience. J Clin Psychol 62(5):551–568

Brody DS 1980 The patient's role in clinical decision-making. Ann Intern Med 93:718–722

Capra F 1982 The Turning Point, science, society, and the rising culture. Bantam Books, Toronto

Coulehan JL, Block MR 2001 The Medical Interview, Mastering Skills for Clinical Practice, fourth edition. FA Davies Company, Philadelphia

Davenport S, Goldberg D, Miller T 1987 How psychiatric disorders are missed during medical consultations. Lancet 2:439–441

Delbanco TL 1992 Enriching the doctor-patient relationship by inviting the patient's perspective. Ann Intern Med 116(5)

Epstein RM, Quill TE, McWhinney IR 1990 Somatization reconsidered: incorporating the patient's experience of illness. Arch Intern Med 159(3):215–222

Freud S 1962 'The anxiety neuroses', in The Standard Edition of the Psychological Works of Sigmund Freud ed. J. Strachey, Hogarth Press, London

Galloway VA, Brodsky Sl 2003 Caring less, doing more: The role of therapeutic detachment with volatile and unmotivated clients, Am J Psychother 57(1)

González-Crussi F 2007 A Short History of Medicine. Random House, New York

Jarvis C 2000 Physical examination and health assessment, third edition. WB Saunders Company, Philadelphia

Knight ZG 2005 The use of the 'corrective emotional experience' and the search for the bad object in psychotherapy. Am J Psychother 59(1)

Langewitz W, Kiss A, Schächinger H 1998 From perception to symptom – from symptom to diagnosis. Somatoform disorders as a communication phenomenon between physician and patient. Schweiz Med Wochenschr 128(7):231–244

Lindlahr H 1975 Philosophy of Natural Therapeutics. CW Daniel Company, UK

Lloyd IR 2006 Messages from the body, a guide to the energetics of health. Naturopathic Publications, Toronto

Lousie C 2007 Systems Principles and Naturopathic Philosophy: The Human Being as a Complex System. Foundations of Naturopathic Medicine Project, Washington

Maynard DW, Heritage J 2005 Conversation analysis, doctor-patient interaction and medical communication. Med Educ 39:428–435

McGee S 2001 Evidence-Based Physical Diagnosis. Saunders, Philadelphia

McWhinney IR 1981 An Introduction to Family Medicine. Oxford University Press, New York

Medalie JH et al 2000 Two physician styles of focusing on the family, their relation to patient outcomes and process of care. J Fam Pract 49(3)

Mehl-Madrona L 1997 Coyote Medicine. Fireside, New York

Morgan WL, Engel GL 1969 The Clinical Approach to the Patient. WB Saunders, Philidelphia

Noyes R, Holt CS, Kathol RG 1995 Somatization. Diagnosis and management. Arch Fam Med 4(9):790–795

Oschman J 2003 Energy Medicine in Therapeutics and Human Performance. Butterworth-Heinemann, Edinburgh

Penson RT, Gu F, Harris S, et al 2007 Hope. Oncologist 12:1105–1113

Pert C 2002 The Wisdom of the Receptors: Neuropeptides, the Emotions, and Bodymind. Advances 18(1):30–35

Platt FW, McMath JC 1979 Clinical hypocompetence: the interview. Ann Intern Med 91:898–902

Rogers C 1961 On Becoming a Person. Mifflin, Boston

Seller RH 2000 Differential Diagnosis of Common Complaints, fourth edition. WB Saunders Company, Philadelphia

Sperry AC 1990 Promoting health and well-being through a sense of connectedness. Frontier Perspectives 1(2):18–20

Weatch R 1972 Updating the Hippocratic Oath. Med Opin 8:56

8

The therapeutic encounter

CHAPTER 9
Physical assessment

The physical assessment follows the holistic intake. The information gathered during the intake provides the subjective view of the patterns of disharmony. The physical assessment provides an objective look at how the patterns have affected the physical health of the patient. Symptoms and diseases are multifactorial, yet they manifest in ways that have a logical pattern and that convey meaning as to the causative factors. The aim of the physical assessment is to correlate the patterns that emerged during the holistic intake with the physical signs and symptoms, to identify the causative factors, and to determine the treatment strategy that is required to restore health.

The human body is an outward display of the internal patterns. These patterns appear on the psychological, functional, and structural aspects of an individual and they always shift together, in varying degrees. For example, you hear it in the words that a patient chooses and how they speak; there are changes on the tongue and in the pulses, in heart rate and breathing patterns, on their face and skin, and in the alignment of the structural body.

Human beings are complex, dynamic, interrelated systems and the physical body displays a single pattern of disharmony in many different ways, in various parts of the body.

There are countless ways of perceiving what is going on with the person who is in front of you and who needs your help and that there are many ways of stimulating healing response (Oshman 2003).

A thorough physical exam includes the assessment of various parts of the patient as each part provides a unique window and highlights a specific function or part of the body. For example, breathing patterns and pulses change in response to acute stressors, whereas the physical structures, alignment of bones, or the movement of toes represent more chronic or ingrained patterns of disharmony. Each assessment method supplements and verifies the others. The manifestation of the same pattern in different parts of the body provides the practitioner with a thorough and more complete pattern of the patient's condition. For each patient, and each symptom pattern a particular window will provide the clearest view. For example, if a patient has symptoms of joint pain, an assessment of posture will often provide a clearer message than the assessment of pulses or the eyes; if a patient has a range of chronic symptoms, the information conveyed in the eyes and the pulses will often provide a clearer view than a postural assessment.

The body provides many windows for reading the symptom patterns and the more windows that a practitioner looks through, the greater the confirmation of the pattern. The windows, or areas of assessment, provide a range of options for each practitioner, based on their unique skill set and areas of interest. The more that a practitioner studies and practices a specific area of assessment, the greater the depth of information they discover. For example, a practitioner who has mastered tongue and pulse diagnosis will be able to assess the subtleties of a patient's disharmony through that one window. A practitioner does not have to be master of all the aspects of assessment. What is helpful is for a practitioner to discover where their strengths lie and to develop them, without losing sight of the value of the other windows. I encourage practitioners, especially young practitioners, to initially assess all areas of the body in order to discover the various ways that human beings have of expressing disharmony.

In order to interpret the symptom patterns in the body, a practitioner needs to have a detailed knowledge of anatomy, physiology, and pathology. They also need an understanding of how the qualities and attributes are manifested physically and how the body functions as a complex, dynamic system. As with all parts of assessment, a practitioner needs to have an open mind, maintain the art of curiosity and intrigue, and be able to recognize that health and disease is a puzzle; the more pieces to the puzzle that a practitioner uncovers, the more complete the picture.

During a naturopathic physical assessment a practitioner conducts a conventional physical exam includes laboratory testing; as well as an assessment of a patient's posture, gait, breathing patterns, tongue and pulse, face, eyes, hands and feet. As there are many books written on the standard conventional physical exam, that information will not be repeated in this book. The emphasis of this chapter is on assessing how the specific attributes and qualities of patterns appear on the physical body.

PHYSICAL STRUCTURE

The physical structure and appearance of a patient is often the first thing that a practitioner observes. This observation provides the practitioner with an indication of the personality and temperament of the patient. The unique qualities that are observed and attributes that they represent can be understood based on the elemental properties discussed in Chapter 5. Figure 9.1 looks at how the elements appear in shape and form in the body.

- *Earth* build is like an oak tree, strong and firm. Body features have a square shape with definite borders, like a square jaw and shoulders, and a thick, short neck. An earth patient is solid, broad, and big-boned.
- *Water* build has more cushioning and softness. There is roundness to the physical features and a stout build. You see more fat throughout the body and a larger chest.
- *Fire* build is muscular and moderate in size. The features are in proportion and the eyes are sharp and prominent. The skin has more of a red tone.
- *Air* build is like a willow tree, flexible and moving. Air bodies tend to be thin, small boned and without a lot muscle or fat, and they may be underdeveloped. Their features tend to be subtle and their color is usually paler.
- *Ether* is a reflection of an individual's presence and vitality regardless of their shape and size.

Observation

Hippocrates introduced the art of clinical observation as the necessary basis for pathologic diagnosis (Hahnemann 1997). Everything that a practitioner observes holds a meaning. Most of what we observe, in every aspect of our life, is interpreted without our conscious input and awareness of the interpretation process. The mind identifies objects by extracting diagnostic visual cues and matching this information to a prototypical, structural

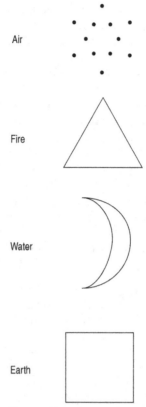

Air

Fire

Water

Earth

Fig 9.1 Shape of the elements. Air – star shape, appears as symptoms that come and go with no precise pattern. Fire – triangle shape, appears as symptoms that have a sharp edge and that are more pointed. Water – moon shape, appears as symptoms that are more rounded and softer. Earth – square shape, appears as symptoms that are hard, firm, square, definite borders.

description stored in memory (Biederman 1987, Bar et al 2001) In order to assess the symptom patterns, it is essential to learn and 'program' energetic pattern correlations for observed (and auditory) clues into the unconscious mental templates that the mind uses for assessment.

The art of assessment is to separate observation from interpretation. For example, a practitioner might observe that a patient's arms are crossed, that their breathing is shallow and rapid, and that their brow is tightened; the interpretation is that a patient is frustrated. But that interpretation might be incorrect. How a practitioner assesses the visual clues of the body depends on their internal 'encyclopedia'. Skilled practitioners are able to pick up detailed information from a patient, sometimes even intuitively, but all information that is picked up should be supported by visual clues.

Many forms of treatment are based on patients becoming aware of how they respond to situations. The more that a practitioner can capture what they are observing the more beneficial it is for the patient. For example, a patient might know that they have anxiety, but they are unaware of the various ways that their body manifests the anxiety, and by becoming aware they have more options and means of treating their condition.

Observation involves having 'soft eyes' and 'open ears'. It recognizes the subtleties as well as the details; the harmony and disharmony that a patient displays. It is about being present in the process, slowing it down, and paying attention. For every aspect of the assessment ask yourself what stands out, what is missing, what seems out of place, and what's different. Before you look for the details, look and listen for the overall pattern that a patient is displaying, such as an overriding sign of excess or deficiency. Most qualities can be caused by a number of different factors; below is an example of the most common causes of the following symptoms:

- sidedness – Yin–Yang pattern
- symptoms located on the periphery – external pattern
- symptoms located in the core or center of the body – internal pattern
- heaviness – excess of water or earth
- light – excess of air, deficiency of earth
- slow – excess of water or earth, deficiency in fire or air
- sharp – excess fire
- cold – excess air or water, deficient in fire or earth
- hot – excess fire or earth, deficient air or water
- oily – excess water
- dry – excess air, fire or earth, deficient water
- rough – excess air
- thick or dense – excess earth
- soft – excess water, or deficiency of earth
- hard – excess earth, or deficiency of water
- cloudy or milky – excess water
- Yin force causes things to contract, to be heavier, and cold. Yin represents the river side of nature. It represents features that are sunken.
- Yang energy represents the mountain side of nature and hence represents features that are raised and have more strength or substance. Yang has an expansive quality.

Palpation

Observation and palpation are inseparable. Any aspect of the body that displays disharmony needs to be assessed in more detail. If a patient has functional symptoms, such as digestive or breathing concerns, it is important to identify if they are related to structural alterations.

Palpation assessment progresses through successive degrees of attenuation from bone to muscles, to fascia, to fluid, to energy fields (Chaitow 1997). The structure of the body governs its function, and function dictates structure and the movement and freedom of motion of every tissue, organ, and cell is needed for efficient working of the body. Palpation determines the degree to which each part of the body is able to move freely and it is used to confirm and expand on any information that is observed.

Every cell, tissue, organ, and structure of the body is linked as a complex dynamic network. There is an intrinsic nature and organizational matrix within the human body, a connection between the skin, muscles, joints, organs, as well as the emotional state of the patient; each one affects the others. There is a flow of fluids and energy throughout the body that nurtures and supports each component. An alternation in any aspect alters the whole.

The role of a practitioner is to observe, assess, touch, feel, and learn from the body. The art of palpation is what a practitioner feels, it cannot be learned in books. It is learning to listen – with your hands – to everything that the body is willing to convey. The art of palpation is a very detailed skill that requires an immense amount of practice and silent attention. I recommend that you explore this skill in more detail by studying the works of authors such as Leon Chaitow, in his book *Palpation Skills*.

The objectives of palpation are to: (Chaitow 1997)

- detect abnormal tissue texture
- evaluate symmetry in the position of structures, both tactically and visually
- detect and assess variations in range and quality of movement during the range, as well as the quality of the end of the range of any movement
- sense the position in space of yourself and the patient being palpated
- detect and evaluate change in the palpated findings, whether these are improving or worsening as time passes.

Palpation also detects changes in energy variations, 'tissue memory', and detects differences in tissue texture and quality in various aspects of the body. It involves correlating a patient's perception of discomfort or disharmony with observational and palpation findings. Palpation provides information as to the qualities of the patterns that are being manifested. For example, muscles overall represent the quality of fire. Too much earth in the fire element shows up as stiffness and increased tone in muscles; a deficiency of earth manifests as atrophy or a lack of normal tone.

Tools such as scans, radiographs and laboratory tests are used by naturopathic doctors and they provide valuable information as to the structural changes in the body, but they do not replace the information that is obtained by observation and palpation.

> Although palpation is commonly thought of as a means of accumulating evidence to be used when coming towards an assessment, diagnostic or prognostic position, there exist situations in many areas of manual palpation where there is only a theoretical division between palpation/assessment and therapeutic activity (Chaitow 1997).

Posture

A patient's posture reveals their sense of inner and outer support, their flexibility, and their openness to external factors. The way a person moves and stands indicates inner characteristics (Mattsson & Mattsson 2002). An aligned posture allows for movement through the full length of the body.

Assessing posture is very important especially when pain and discomfort with movement is a concern, or when you observe structural changes. Posture is the result of the over use, misuse, or abuse of underlying structures of the body, and their respective alignment and positioning both right to left and front to back over time. It is affected by the size and strength of the bones –

an earth quality; the fluid within the joint spaces – a water quality; the muscles that attach to the bone – a fire quality; the ease and freedom of movement – an air quality; and the desire to take up space – an ether quality.

Misalignment of posture occurs because of injuries and habitual patterns, such as crossing the legs, or tilting the head while talking on the phone, or an imbalanced stance. Postural assessment determines how posture affects the functioning of the body, and it explores the impact of habits and injuries on physical structure.

When assessing posture, look at the body from the front, the back, and the sides, both when a patient is standing and when they are lying down (Fig. 9.2). It is easiest to see the key features of posture when a patient is wearing as few clothes as is reasonable. A gravity board, plumb line, and grid wall are the easiest ways to properly identify and measure the differences in the posture alignment. Initially assess your patient in as relaxed and natural state as possible. You are looking for how they normally stand and how their weight is distributed. Next have them stand with their heels exactly in line and square to a real or imaginary plumb line running down the center of the body from the head to the feet. The following are the main patterns that are displayed in a postural assessment:

- *Lateral or medial deviation.* The hands, arms, legs, and feet are body parts that most easily demonstrate lateral or medial deviation which indicate external and internal patterns, respectively. Lateral deviation is when the body parts are pointed or positioned away from the center line, such as patient who stands with their left leg externally rotated (refer to Fig. 5.2). Lateral deviation or movement is due to a patient either pushing away from themselves or being pulled by external situations. Medial deviation is when the body parts are pointed or positioned toward the center line, such as a patient who sits with their knees internally rotated (refer to Fig. 5.3). Medial deviation or movement is due to a patient pulling inward or avoiding external situations.
- *Right to left difference.* Any difference right to left is a reflection of a Yin–Yang pattern. You often notice one side of the body that is wider and has a more pronounced muscle mass. It is not uncommon for people's hands and feet to be aligned differently right to left. The presence of other signs and symptoms will reveal whether this is a natural state for a patient or a sign of disharmony.
- *Top to bottom differences* relate to differences from the hips to the feet, and from the shoulders to the hips on either side of the body. For some people, the difference is all on one side. For others, there is a difference in the upper body on one side and the lower body on the other side; their body is twisted. The upper body has more to do with the interaction between oneself and others. The lower body is more about moving through life.
- *Front to back difference.* A difference front to back relates to a patient's center of gravity and by observing the distribution of weight that is in front of the center line and how much is behind it. The front of the body is Yin and represents the sensory aspects of the body; the back of the body is Yang and represents the motor aspects. When the weight is shifted more forward or backward it will often have a corresponding Yin–Yang pattern.

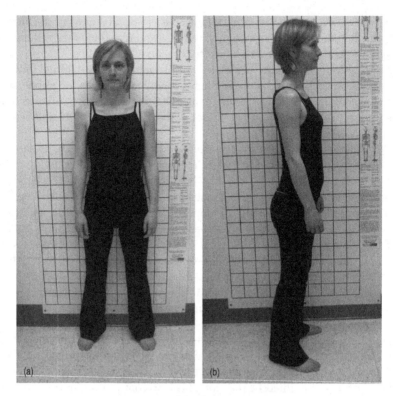

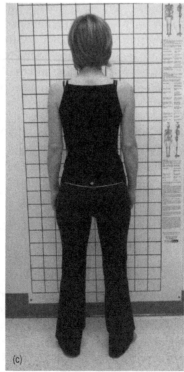

Fig 9.2 Postural assessment. (a) From the front; (b) from the side; (c) from the back.

The alignment of posture front to back is also indicative of underlying functional changes in the body. For example,

If the head is pulled back, the movement of the neck is restricted and the chest is more fixed and immobile, which means restrictions in exploration and perception of the surroundings. Carriage coincides with a stiff way of viewing the world – rules are followed categorically, fantasy is an obstacle and rigid working-style is favoured (Mattsson & Mattsson 2002).

GAIT ASSESSMENT

A patient's gait provides information of how the physical body moves within space. It shows how the different parts of the body flow together and the symmetry right to left and top to bottom. Imbalances in gait also highlight structural or functional concerns.

When a patient walks their posture is often different than when they stand: for example they lead with a specific part of the body. If there is a specific part of the body that is leading, look for the symbolism of that body part to provide information on the pattern they are displaying.

When a patient displays an aligned posture and good balance in their gait it implies that they have the ability and strength to preserve the alignment between their head and pelvis. This is important as the center of gravity is in the pelvis.

The arms follow the trunk, giving equilibrium and emphasizing pace. The gaze is directed straight ahead, the head and neck move freely in the vertical line, the eyes and ears readily incorporating necessary information. This way of walking is open and grounded; there are few restrictions (Mattsson & Mattsson 2002).

When assessing a patient's gait initially do so when they are unaware, such as when they are walking to the practitioner's office. As soon as you bring a patient's awareness to their walk it often changes. A patient compensates or exaggerates a feature that they are aware is out of balance. Also, assess their walk in the gait that is most comfortable for them, their natural state. Then ask them to speed it up and slow it down. Notice how they handle the change and what changes in their posture. How a patient walks displays certain qualities and characteristics that relate to the elements and to Yin and Yang.

- *Earth* walk is slow, steady, and heavy. It indicates a person who stands firmly on the ground and who expresses stability and firmness.
- *Water* walk is flowing and continuous, like a gentle stroll.
- *Fire* walking is fast, intense, and with a clear direction.
- *Air* walk is quick with frequent changes in direction.
- The quality of *ether* is seen as the ease and ability of walking overall.
- The quality of *Yin–Yang* is seen when there is a difference between the right and left sides of the body or the top and bottom of the body. For example, you might see that the right arm swings more freely than the left. Or that the legs and hips are very rigid, yet the upper body is more relaxed.

ASSESSMENT OF JOINTS

It is common for patients to have pain or discomfort around joints, as joints are responsible for movement of the structural body. Overall joints represent the qualities of space – ether – that is the freedom to move through life. As ether is the element from which all other elements are derived, the movement of the joints and the location of joint symptoms bring in all the other elements. The joints located in the core of the body, the spine, relate to the freedom of movement that a patient feels with respect to themselves, and their ability to be themselves. The movement of the peripheral joints relates more to the interaction between a patient and their external surroundings. The joints on the upper body also have a corresponding joint on the lower body; for example the elbows and the knees are both air joints, the wrists and ankles are both water joints. The joints on the top of the body refer more to acute or current situations, the joints on the lower aspect of the body often relate more to chronic situations or patterns.

Each joint has a corresponding symbolic meaning, for example the shoulders symbolize giving and receiving, hips symbolize moving forward. The elbow and knee correlate with the qualities and characteristics of air element; the wrist and ankle correlate with the water element (see Fig. 9.3).

- The quality of *earth* impacts movement of the joints as it relates to structure and support. An excess of earth appears as guarding, stiffness, or inability to move; a deficiency of earth appears as weakness or lack of strength.
- An excess of *water* impacts joint movement through the presence or absence of fluid and often manifests as swelling or inflammation.
  A deficiency of water results in a loss of fluid in the joint space.
  A water imbalance is also apparent when there is a cogwheel aspect to the movement that is, the movement isn't smooth – it starts and stops.

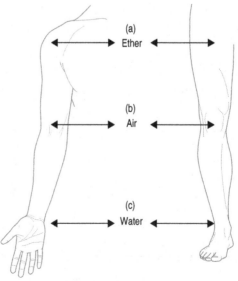

Fig 9.3 Peripheral jonts. (a) Ether joints; (b) air joints; (c) water joints.

- An excess of *fire* results in redness and heat and is one of the main causes of pain. Restlessness in muscles is an indication of excess fire. Muscles are a manifestation of the fire element. Balanced fire is seen in the tone and structure of the muscles themselves.
- The *air* element controls the nervous system. A lack of nervous impulse for the muscles to move indicates an imbalance in the air element, as in the feeling of 'pins and needles', random movements, or twitching.
- *Yang* energy controls the movement of the extensor muscles. An excess of Yang, for example, would manifest as contraction or issues with respect to the extensor muscles. You might also find an area around a joint that was intensely hot and aggravating. The qualities of heat and contraction are also Yang in nature.
- *Yin* energy controls the movement of the flexor muscles. The qualities of cold and expansion are Yin in nature. An example of excess Yin would be when the muscles are lax or weak, or there is a concern around the flexion of the muscles.

BREATHING

Breathing is the first thing you do when you are born and your last breath indicates death. The full potential of breathing is the integration of the body, mind, and spirit; it is a process of experiencing, expressing, and contemplating life.

> *The function of breathing is said to represent a bridge between the conscious and unconscious – breathing can be controlled by our will, but mostly we breathe reflexively (Mattsson & Mattsson 2002).*

Breathing is directly affected by what you are thinking and can affect thinking itself. It is not only essential to life, it is a reflection of life.

Inhalation is an active process where air is brought into the body; exhalation is a passive process where carbon dioxide is released. There is a rhythmic movement between breathing in and breathing out that affects every aspect of an individual. This ebb and flow pattern of contraction, relaxation, and resting is one of the energetic waves of life.

Breathing is quite easy to observe and palpate and carries with it a lot of information. The volume, speed, consistency, location of breath, origin of breath, frequency, phrasing (difference between the inhalation and exhalation), texture (smooth and even or jerky and uneven), depth (deep or shallow) and quality (pneumatic or labored), all provide information about an individual's health on the psychological, functional, and structural levels.

When patients are dealing with stress, of any type, the initial response of the body, often unconscious, is for the breath to become rapid and shallow. For example, the term 'anxiety' has its linguistic root in the Latin word *angustio*, which corresponds to suffocation. Likewise, when a person feels anxious it will feel as if breathing is obstructed (Mattsson & Mattsson 2002).

The qualities of breathing can be broken down into inhalation, exhalation, and the rest period as described in Table 9.1.

Breathing overall is an air element, yet the influences, excess and deficiency of all the elements affect breath. What you are assessing with breathing is the

Physical assessment

9

Table 9.1 Breathing

Energy group	Inhalation	Exhalation	Rest period
Purpose	Experience life	Express life 'letting go'	Contemplate life 'stillness'
Key function in the body	Oxygenates blood	Eliminates cellular waste and maintains the acid–base balance of the blood	Homeodynamic state, integration of the body, mind, and emotions
Nervous system	*Sympathetic* fight or flight, increases heart rate, decreases digestive action and activity	*Central nervous system* regulates and monitors physiology of body	*Parasympathetic* meditative state relaxes body after stress, decreases heart rate, increases digestion, energy conserving
Current	*Spiral* quality of energy and movement, warmth, building and healing	*Long lines* carry energy of mind into the body and govern the senses, cleansing	*East/west* intercommunication and binding, neutral feedback pattern relating the periphery to the core
Principles	Positive	Negative	Neutral
Yin–Yang	Yin	Yang	Neutral
Movement	Direction	Completion	Dispersing
Element	Fire	Water	Air and ether

freedom of the air element to move among and within the other elements. The following is how the energetic patterns manifest in breath.

- The quality of *earth* is seen in the slowness and depth of the breath.
- The quality of *water* is seen in a patient's ability to exhale, to let go. It manifests in the flow of the breath. It appears in the consistency and rhythmic nature of the breathing pattern.
- The quality of *fire* is seen in the inhalation. It is the impulse to breathe itself. Inhalation has to do with experiencing life, having the impulse to take in from the outside. Excess fire in the breath manifests as a breath that is too rapid.
- The quality of *air* is seen in the overall breathing pattern. Breath brings in prana or life energy. The act of breathing is responsible for moving energy throughout the body.
- *Ether* is represented in the body's ability to breathe itself, having the space and will to breathe. Ether represents the overall quality of the breath.

Steps to assessing breathing patterns

Assessing breathing patterns involves conventional methods, such as auscultation and radiographs to rule in and rule out specific diseases, such as asthma, bronchitis, pneumonia, and lung pathologies. There are many factors that can disrupt normal breathing patterns and assessing the qualities

THE ENERGETICS OF HEALTH

184

of how a patient breathes provides another layer of information that is helpful in determining the causative factors and in deciding on the treatment strategy that is the most appropriate. For example, a sigh is a deep and shallow breath. It is a symptom of fatigue, depression, or grief. The word 'to sigh' means 'to lament, mourn over'. Yawning is a sign of drowsiness, dullness, or boredom. It has the quality of earth. Anxiety, on the other hand, causes rapid, shallow breaths. It is often associated with fire or air imbalances.

The following is a guide for assessing the patterns of breathing:

1. *Observation.* What was the first thing that you noticed about a patient's breathing? Was it the sound or movement?
2. *Visual.* When a patient inhales is the chest expanding or the belly expanding? Do the scapulae move appropriately and equally? What is the difference in comfort that a patient experiences between the inhalation and exhalation? How rapid is the breathing? How does the breath change in response to different parts of the conversation, or to different stimuli?
3. *Auditory.* Normally you don't hear a patient breathe. Sound usually indicates constriction or the act of taking a deeper breath than usual. What is the frequency and severity of the sound?
4. *Palpation.* When palpating for lung expansion, pay attention to both sides simultaneously. Where does the breath stop? What is different right to left? How does the spinal column and body move in response to the breath? It is easiest to feel the breath by firmly placing your hands on the posterior aspect of the ribs, just under the diaphragm. Have your patient take deep breaths and feel what happens under your hands. Watch the spinal column as your patient breathes. Are there aspects of the spinal column that don't expand?

TONGUE ASSESSMENT

The tongue is the organ of taste and speech, and it is a window into the inner body, especially the digestive system (Maciocia 1998). It is an essential diagnostic tool of naturopathic, Ayurvedic and Chinese medical assessments. Tongue diagnosis, like pulse diagnosis, takes time and experience to master. The tongue conveys a lot about the inner status of the body and once a practitioner has learned to interpret the signs appropriately, it is a clear indication of the underlying disharmony. The more you look at patients' tongues with curiosity and notice the nuances, differences, and changes that can occur, the more you will be able to read this wonderful road map. The following provides an overview of the key features and what they indicate. I encourage you to study tongue diagnosis in more detail as you develop beyond the basics.

The tongue is viewed from the tip to the root (see Fig. 9.4). The tip of the tongue relates to the upper body, the lungs, and the heart. The middle aspect of the tongue relates to the area between the diaphragm and umbilicus and it represents the stomach and the spleen. The root of the tongue relates to the area between the umbilicus and pelvis as well as, the liver and gallbladder. It represents the kidneys, bladder, colon, and reproductive organs (Maciocia 1998).

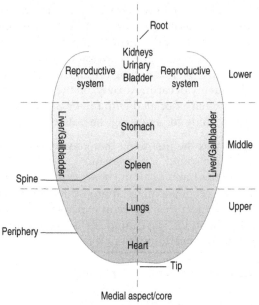

Fig 9.4 Anatomical zones of the tongue. (a) Upper – the area above the diaphragm; (b) middle – the area between the diaphragm and waist; (c) lower – the area below the waist.

Naturopathic, Ayurvedic and Chinese medicine recognize that organs have a structural function, and an energetic function. Different emotions are held in different organs, the organs continually communicate to each other, and they provide fuel for each other. Imbalances seen on the tongue represent the energetics qualities of the organs, more so than the physical structure of the organs. For example, seeing congestion in the area of the liver on the tongue does not mean that liver tests will show any functional changes. It means that the energetics of the liver is currently in disharmony. It is very common for patterns to manifest on the tongue and pulse prior to them manifesting as a physical symptom or prior to laboratory tests indicating disease.

There are four main aspects to tongue diagnosis: the body color, body shape, coating and moisture. When examining the tongue, the following guidelines will ensure the best findings (Maciocia 1998):

- use natural sunlight
- ask the patient to extend their tongue as much as possible, but avoid excessive force
- have patients extend their tongue only for about 15–20 seconds; if it is extended for a longer period of time, the tongue will become more red and distort the true findings
- the consumption of coffee, wine, and highly colored foods and sweets affect tongue color; advise patients not to consume these foods prior to the examination
- tobacco, medications and antibiotics might distort the findings on the tongue.

Table 9.2	Tongue body color (Lloyd 2005, Maciocia 1989)
Characteristic	*Indications*
Pale	Yang, blood deficiency or an excess of Yin or cold
Red	Yang excess, Yin deficiency or too much internal heat, red raised papillae indicates a fire quality
Purple	Stasis of blood, heat or energy
Blue	Excess internal coldness, blood stasis

Body color

The body color of the tongue (Table 9.2) reflects the key underlying pattern in the body. It indicates the presence of Yin or Yang patterns. When a patient's subjective or symptom presentation is contradictory, as it often is, the color of the tongue body is the most reliable sign and always points to the true condition. The reason for this is that the body color of the tongue is relatively unaffected by short-term events and recent changes in a person's life (Maciocia 1998). The tongue's body color is also the most important indicator of improvement or decline in a patient's condition. The normal color of the body of the tongue is pink.

Body shape

The shape of the tongue (Table 9.3) relates to the structure and size of the tongue. It reflects the quality of excess and deficiency, the presence of cracks and ulcers, the stiffness or subtleness of the tongue, and the movement. It also shows signs of a Yin–Yang pattern (Maciocia 1998).

Table 9.3	Tongue body shape (Lloyd 2005, Maciocia 1989)
Characteristic	*Indications*
Thin	Deficiency state, chronic
Swollen	Excess state
Stiff	Excess state. The body is guarded or held in a contracted state – an earth excess quality
Flaccid	Deficiency of body fluids
Cracked	Either due to a deficiency in fluids, an excess of heat, or an excess of air
Quivering	A deficiency state. An inability of the inner body to deal with all different energetic influences or a state of overwhelm due to external or environmental factors
Scalloped or tooth marks	Spleen Qi deficiency from a Chinese point of view. Indicates an inability to digest or poor assimilation (either of nutrients or 'life')

Physical assessment

Table 9.4 Tongue coating (Lloyd 2005, Maciocia 1989)	
Characteristic	*Indications*
Thick	Presence of pathogenic factor or an internal toxin
Absent	Overall deficiency pattern, often seen with chronic illness
White	Cold, water, Yin condition
Yellow	Heat, fire, Yang condition
Gray and black	Extreme cold or extreme heat, for example sepsis

Tongue coating

Examining the coating on a tongue is done systematically from the tip to the root, examining each aspect separately and as part of the whole (Table 9.4). The coating on the tongue reflects hot and cold, the presence of a pathogen, internal toxins, and reflects the progression and location of disease. The tongue coating varies in thickness, color, texture, and general appearance. The darker, thicker, and more widespread the coating, the greater the presence of a pathogen or the more the disease has progressed. The normal coating of a tongue is thin and white. In a healthy state, you can see the pink body color through the coating.

Tongue moisture

The moisture on a tongue indicates the presence of body fluids (Table 9.5). Normally a tongue will appear slightly moist. Any deviation from this indicates a deficiency or excess of water or body fluids (Maciocia 1998).

Table 9.5 Tongue moisture (Lloyd 2005, Maciocia 1989)	
Characteristic	*Indications*
Dry	Heat, fire, excess Yang, or deficiency of Yin; also dry and cracked is an air quality
Moist	Either excess water, Yin, or deficiency of Yang. This represents an inability of the body to move fluids throughout; if extreme can also indicate dampness
Sticky/ slippery	Retention of dampness or phlegm. The fluids are stuck and built up in an area as seen in excess water/earth pattern

PULSE DIAGNOSIS

Pulse diagnosis is an integral part of most traditional systems of medicine (Fig. 9.5). It provides a clear window into the pulsating waves of the body as the health of the organs can be felt in the different pulses. In Chinese medicine pulse taking has been used as one of the most important diagnostic tools for over 2000 years and is considered one of the most valuable of all the devices to which a physician can resort (Kuriyama 1999). Pulse diagnosis is subtle and complex. It receives information through kinesthetic, visual, and intuitive channels. This information is then evaluated using the

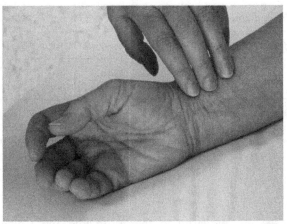

Fig 9.5 Examining the pulses. Patient's arm is extended and relaxed with the palm facing upward. Practitioner's fire finger (middle) is placed beside and proximal to the styloid process of the radius, on the radial artery. The air finger is placed distal to the fire finger, and the water finger is proximal.

knowledge of physiology, energetics, and the information received from the patient.

Conventional diagnosis often refers to the identification of disease after it has manifested. Assessment tools such as pulse diagnosis allow a practitioner to monitor the stages of health and disease throughout the process. The wave of the pulses shifts in response to subtle and profound energetic changes. For example, exercising, eating, and arguing, all temporarily change the pulses. The pulses indicate how the body fluids or organ systems are maintaining their dynamic balance. Chronic illness has a more profound impact on pulses and can dampen the normal acute changes in pulse.

When examining the pulses it is best to do so at least 30 minutes after a meal or exercise (Lad 1998). The practitioner and the patient must be relaxed to accurately feel the pulses. The radial artery often is used as the point to tune into the inner body. The practitioner's air, fire, and water fingers are used to sense the pulse. The air finger of the practitioner's right hand is placed in the distal aspect of the radial artery, at the wrist crease of the patient's left arm. The fire finger is placed parallel to the air finger, and the water finger is placed on the proximal aspect, next to the fire finger. The practitioner's left hand is applied to the patient's right arm in the same fashion. The air finger is always distal, fire finger in the middle, and water finger proximal (Hammer 2005).

Each holistic system of medicine that uses pulse diagnosis has its own unique way of reading the pulses (Table 9.6). There is similarity, but the language and the window for each is different. Each approach will lead a practitioner to the same conclusions, once they have mastered the art of pulse taking. Assessing the pulse provides insight and information the more it is used. It is a skill that grows in precision and depth of understanding all the time. When a practitioner is initially exploring the pulses as a form of diagnosis, it is best to look at the overall picture, the patterns that are the most overt. Once you have felt 1000 pulses and have a concept of the subtleties that can exist, it is valuable to expand your technical knowledge by studying Ayurvedic or Chinese medicine. This book will provide a starting point for pulse diagnosis.

Physical assessment

189

Table 9.6 Pulse diagnosis (Lloyd 2005, Maciocia 1989, Hammer 2005)

Practitioner's finger position	Ayurvedic window	Traditional Chinese medicine window	
		Organs (patient's right hand)	Organs (patient's left hand)
Distal/air finger	Ether/air (Vata)	Lung	Heart
Middle/fire finger	Fire/water (Pitta)	Stomach/Spleen	Liver
Proximal/water finger	Water/earth (Kapha)	Kidney Yang	Kidney Yin

You can see the similarity in the Ayurvedic and Chinese medicine approach. The distal pulse represents the upper 1/3 of the body, the area above the diaphragm. It represents the elements of ether and air. The lung and the heart are both air organs. The middle pulse represents the middle thorax, the area between the diaphragm and the umbilicus. It represents the element of fire primarily. The stomach, spleen, and liver are all fire organs. The proximal pulse represents the lower aspect of the thorax, the area between the umbilicus and the pelvic area. It represents the elements of water and earth (Lad 1998).

What is also common is that both Ayurvedic and Chinese medicine feel the pulse on three levels; superficial, middle, and deep (Zhen 1985, Lad 1998). The superficial level is felt on the surface with a light touch. Use moderate pressure to feel the middle pulse. You need to press quite hard to feel the deep pulse. The superficial pulse represents the most outward aspect of the body, the middle pulse represents the presence of the pulse in the middle aspect of the body and the deep pulse represents the presence of the pulse deep within the body.

The pulse must be felt for at least five beats at each level to establish a clear pattern (Zhen 1985). A normal pulse is between four to five beats per breath and the quality is smooth, elastic, present, and flowing (Hammer 2005). The following provides a guide to how pulses manifest based on specific patterns.

- *External condition.* Assessment of the pulse in the superficial position is used to assess for the presence of disease due to external conditions. When the pulse is floating the body has shifted the energy to the upper body or to the periphery to help fight off the pathogen. For example, this often is felt in the lung position at the onset of a cold or flu.
- *Internal condition.* When the pulses are deep and only felt with heavy pressure it indicates the presence of an internal condition and often a chronic condition. The blocked energy is sitting deep within the body and energy is focused at that level.
- *Excess.* A pattern of excess creates a pulse that is full and faster than five beats per respiration. It will feel strong, long, and thick. It often is due to excess fire or heat or Yang excess.
- *Deficiency.* A pattern of deficiency creates a pulse that feels empty. The pulse feels big, soft and difficult to feel. There isn't a lot of energy in the

wave pulsation. The pulse might also be slow, short, and thin, or might collapse when you apply pressure. It often is due to a Yin or cold condition or a chronic condition in any organ.

FACE AND SPECIAL SENSES

The face is the most exposed aspect of a patient and it is the main visual aspect that is used to identify someone. The face is very expressive and it not only shows who a patient is, but also shows what has happened to them (Bridges 2004).

Many mental states are displayed as clear as daylight on the face, as virtual print-outs of internal experiences, simply waiting to be read by an observer (Ohashi 1991; Baron-Cohen et al 1997). The belief that the face reveals information about underlying character cuts across national, cultural, and geographical boundaries and this belief has been supported for over 2500 years (Mason et al 2006) For example, Aristotle noted that

Men with small foreheads are fickle, whereas if they are rounded or bulging out the owners are quick-tempered. Straight eyebrows indicate softness of disposition, those that curve out toward the temples, humour and dissimulation. The staring eye indicates impudence, the wrinkling indecision. Large and outstanding eyes indicate a tendency to irrelevant talk or chattering (Liggett 1974).

The face is a complex web of muscles that are able to reveal subtle changes in mood, temperament, and in physical health.

When assessing the face, it is important to be cognizant of cultural differences and the impact of external factors, such as reconstructive surgery and botox injections. Studying the characteristics of the face and assigning personality characteristics to the findings is known as physiognomy. What studies in physiognomy have shown is that for basic emotions the whole face is more informative than either the eyes or the mouth, whereas for complex mental states, seeing the eyes alone is more informative than the mouth on its own, or the whole face (Baron-Cohen et al 1997). Also different emotions appear more prominently on different aspects of the face. For example, the expression of happy emotions was more prominent in the face; while the emotions of fear and surprise were more apparent in the eyes (Hanawalt 1994).

The head is the sensory center of the body. The sense organs provide an entrance to larger internal systems; for example, the mouth opens to the digestive tract, the nose to the respiratory system, the eyes to the optic nerve, the mind, and the brain, and the ears to hearing (Ohashi 1991). Congestion in any of the organ systems results in corresponding congestion in the areas that relate to them.

When assessing the face, start out by looking at the face overall (Fig. 9.6). Notice what stands out the most, the most prominent feature. Observe the harmony between different components of the face and between right and left sides. Each side of the face often reveals a different story, for example it is common for males to have a larger left side and women a larger right side (Hardie et al 2005). This pattern corresponds to the Yin–Yang pattern.

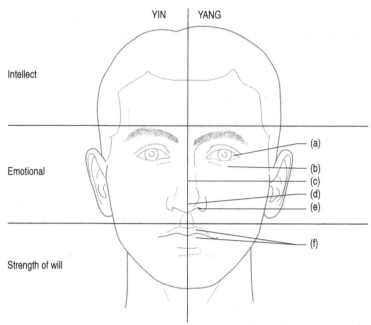

Fig 9.6 Overall face. Right side of the face is Yin, left side is Yang. Center represents the core, the midline of the body and the spine, which encompasses the qualities of ether and earth. (a) Eyes – mind, and nervous system (air); (b) under eyes – kidneys (water); (c) bridge of nose – a patient's inner strength (earth); (d) round part of nose – heart (air); (e) nostrils – lungs (air); (f) mouth – digestion (fire) and nourishment (water).

Make note of the overall observations that you pick up from the face and then concentrate on the individual features that stand out the most. The structure, shape, and look of the face reveal characteristics of a patient. For example, a square strong jaw line is an expression of earth. Rounded, plumb features are a quality of water. A face that is red and intense is expressing more fire. Fine, soft features are seen more in air people. The vitality of a patient is an expression of their ether and it is seen in the overall look and sense of being alive that someone conveys.

Eyes

It is through the expression in the eyes that a patient reveals their state of mind and their innermost feelings.

If the eyes are clear and have glitter, they indicate that the mind and the Essence are in a good state of vitality. If the eyes are rather dull or clouded, the mind is disturbed (Maciocia 1989).

The eyes reveal the state of the nervous system and tension that a patient is holding. They are the most expressive part of the face, especially for complex emotions and often are referred to as the window to the soul (Nummenmaa 1964). For example, if a patient has something to hide they might avoid looking directly at you. If someone is completely open and wishes to get to know you better, often they look straight into your eyes. Cultural differences are very important when exploring the eyes. For example, with native Americans who are raised traditionally, looking someone directly in the eye, especially an elder is a sign of disrespect, whereas for many cultures it represents honesty and attentiveness.

The eyes are the receivers of all visual stimuli the perception of sight and the processing of the information is done by the brain. When there is an endless stream of visual stimuli, the processing aspects are not allowed to rest, for example when constantly surrounded by too much light and constantly bombarded with signage and advertising or television. Computer work and watching television is not only hard on the eyes because of the electromagnetic rays, it also keeps the eyes fixed and limits the movement of the eyes (Jones 1991). To maintain healthy eyes it is important for the muscles to be able to relax, for the visual input to subside, and for the eyes to regenerate on a daily basis. Near and far sightedness is a reflection of the elasticity of the lens of the eye and the flexibility and movement of the eye muscles. The eyes also relate to a patient's life vision and as such, a patient unsure of their future might be near sighted.

The eyes are typically assessed according to their position and how open they are. Each feature of the eyes reveals different qualities (Fig. 9.7). For example:

- *Their placement*. The more lateral the placement of the eyes, the more a patient's vision is influenced or focused on their external world. Eyes that are more medial and closer together represent vision that is more internally focused and self-aware.
- *Their size and shape*. Eyes that have an air quality are smaller, dry, and often have a dull color; fire eyes are moderate in size, and have a focused and penetrating quality; water eyes are large, round, and romantic looking; earth eyes are smaller, still, and more deep set.
- *Their stillness*. The ability of a patient to hold their gaze is reflected in the stillness of the eyes. Flickering or twitches of the eyes suggest either a state of excess or deficiency typically in the air element. If the flickering is more on the right it indicates a yang imbalance, if on the left, a yin imbalance. Stillness is also a quality of ether (content with life) and earth (focused on details); a lot of random movement is an indication of excess air.
- *The area under the eyes relates to the kidney*. If there is an imbalance in the water element it often shows up in the area under the eyes.

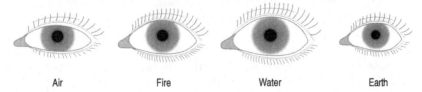

| Air | Fire | Water | Earth |

Fig 9.7 The eyes. (a) Air quality – small, dry, blink frequently; (b) fire quality – moderate size, sharp; (c) water quality – large, moist; (d) earth quality – smaller, slow moving.

Ears

The ears are the most important and revealing aspect of a patient's inner strength. They indicate a patient's inner nature and are associated with their essence, vitality, and constitutional strength: the ether element. They relate to the willingness to listen to others and to one's higher self. Ears are one of the most distinguishing features of the face and unlike other features, they seldom change shape as the face develops; they often only change in size.

The quality of the cartilage of the ear was originally used as one of the predictors of long life. When you grasp the ear between the thumb and forefinger and bend the ear forward (Fig. 9.8) if the cartilage is too stiff it indicates increased internal tension, a normal amount of flexibility and tensile strength indicates a strong constitution, and if the ear is flimsy, thin, or transparent it indicates a weak constitution (Bridges 2004).

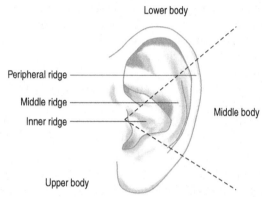

Fig 9.8 Ears. Lower body – below the umbilicus. Middle body – between the diaphragm and umbilicus. Upper body – above the diaphragm Peripheral ridge – circulatory and excretory systems. Middle ridge – nervous system. Inner ridge – digestive and respiratory systems.

The different features of the ears reveal the following:

- *Placement.* Ears are normally positioned level with the eyes and the crease of the mouth. When the top of the ear is higher, then the patient will likely have more air qualities, i.e. be intellectual; when lower the patient will likely have more fire and water qualities, i.e. emotional and nurturing of others.
- *Size and prominence.* Large prominent ears indicate a strong constitution, especially if the ear lobes are large and firm. Large ears also reveal a patient who is more of a risk taker, engages more with life, and enjoys listening to others. Small ears reveal a patient that is more cautious, careful, and often fearful. They tend to be more introverted, they listen to themselves and have a more limited perspective.
- *Shape.* The lower part of the ear represents the upper part of the body, the middle part represents the middle part of the body, and the upper part of the ear represents the lower part of the body. The peripheral ridge indicates the health of the circulatory and excretory systems, the middle ridge the nervous system, and the inner ridge indicates the digestive and respiratory system.
- *Distance from the head.* The angle between the ear and the head shows the harmonious balance between a patient's physical and mental status, and normally this angle should be less than 30 degrees. Ears that tend to stick out reveal people who seek new experiences from the external world and can easily become over-stimulated with external information. When a

patient has ears that are very flat and are close to the head it indicates a person who is less inclined to listen to a lot of external information, they are good listeners, and they are comfortable with their own thoughts. When a patient has ear lobes that are attached it indicates that they have a narrower view of life and prefer solitary work or have a solitary focus.

- *Markings.* Creases, markings, cysts, or anything else on the ear lobe reveals an imbalance in the particular part of the body that area represents. For example, a crease in the lower ear lobe is often associated with heart conditions.

Nose

The nose is the bridge linking the higher self and the physical self. It is used to smell and is one of the instruments of breathing. The bridge of the nose represents the spine or core, the round edge is associated with the heart, and the nostrils are associated with the lungs (Fig. 9.9); hence the nose mirrors the elements of earth (core and sense of smell) and air (heart and lungs) (Kushi 1983; Ohashi 1991). At birth the nose is not fully developed because a patient's ego or core is not developed. The following are the key features to observe about the nose:

- *Size.* A small nose often reflects someone who has a weaker or not fully developed sense of self, a tendency to go along with other people's wishes and to be influenced by others. A large and strong nose reveals someone who is confident and has a strong, often unyielding, sense of self.
- *Position.* If the nose veers off to the right or left it indicates a Yin–Yang quality. Lateral changes in the nose are often due to weakness in the spine or external influences that have affected one's ego. A patient that relies on a sense of self from others has a broader nose, whereas a straighter nose indicates more self confidence.

Physical assessment

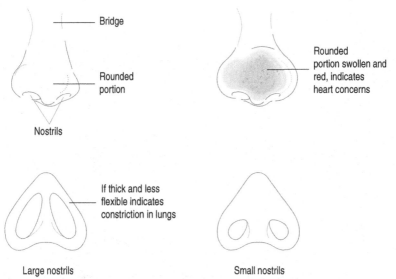

Fig 9.9 Nose. Bridge – core strength/spine, which relates to earth qualities. Rounded portion – heart, which relates to air qualities. Nostrils – lungs, which relates to air qualities.

• *Nostrils.* Nostrils are responsible for drawing in the breath of life. They are involved in breathing and represent the relationship between the subconscious and conscious mind. Nostrils are associated with the lungs and lungs represent the body's ability to take in the life force or Qi. Wide flaring nostrils indicate large lungs, an excess of air, or a Yang excess. If the nostrils are thickened it might indicate tension in the lungs. (The lungs and large intestine are paired organs according to Chinese medicine and hence the lungs become congested when the large intestine cannot eliminate. To treat congestion of the lungs it is often necessary to treat the bowels.) If the round aspect of the nose is red or inflamed it might indicate a weakness or inflammation in the heart. When the nostrils face outward it indicates that the patient will react to the actions of others. Inward nostrils reflect someone who is a self-starter, one who is not easily swayed by others.

Mouth

The mouth is related to the digestive tract, it is also considered a sexual organ, and it is the aspect of the body involved in verbal communication. Even non-verbally it is a significant form of expression and, apart from the eyes, people remember actors' and actresses' mouths more than any other facial feature. Together with the eyes, the mouth conveys personality most immediately, betraying sympathetic or aversion vibrations, coldness and warmth. The normal width of a mouth equals the distance between the pupils of the eyes (Ohashi 1991). The following are the key features to observe about the mouth (Fig. 9.10):

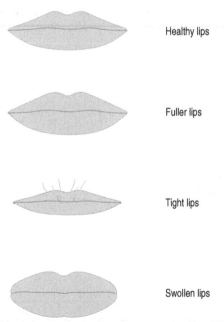

Healthy lips

Fuller lips

Tight lips

Swollen lips

Fig 9.10 Mouth. Healthy lips – evenly developed, moist, pink color. Fuller lips – more water qualities, generous, sensual, kind, more positive. Tight lips – less water qualities, more reserved, tendency to be negative. Swollen lips – indicates distention of digestive tract.

- *Size*. When the mouth is wide it is a sign of an expanded intestinal tract, and digestive trouble (Kushi 1983). A small mouth reveals less of a water influence, and indicates a patient who is less outgoing and often is more cautious.
- *Open or closed*. People whose mouth often is open, even as adults, reveal a lack of the qualities in earth. They tend to have lower self esteem and leave decision-making to others. When a patient's mouth is half open it reveals more of an affectionate, sociable, and dynamic nature. When the mouth is always closed, the lips tight and corners turned down, it is a sign of excess earth and often reflects someone who is gloomy, has a pessimistic nature, or someone who is prone to seeing more of the negative side of life.
- *Lips*. If the lips are swollen they often indicate inflammation in the digestive system and often weak nutrient assimilation. If the lips are not swollen or distended it indicates a strong digestion. Full lips reveal an affectionate and vital nature, a patient who is able to sympathize and share others feelings. If the lips protrude, it is a sign that sometimes this patient will go out of their way to appeal to others. Thin 'hollow' lips often indicate a deficiency state that is affecting the digestive system. Ideally the corners of the mouth are turned up which indicates inner optimism and a positive outlook. A down-turn represents disappointment, and one up and one down corner indicates that a person feels one thing and shows another (Bridges 2004).

TEETH

The teeth relate to a patient's constitution and they relate to the structure aspect of the body which is an earth quality. The teeth display different corresponding patterns within the body, for example there are 32 teeth and 32 vertebrae and a patient's ability to chew depends on the straightness of the spine; tension in the back is often expressed as gritting the teeth (Ohashi 1991). Also, every organ system has a corresponding tooth (Table 9.7) and it often is found that there are problems with a tooth, such as cavities or infection, when there is an imbalance in that organ.

SKIN

Skin is the largest organ of the body and it is an organ of elimination for all internal organ systems. It is able to express many different qualities and various emotional states. 'The skin is the boundary separating the Self from the external world; thus it participates both in the subjective and the objective reality (Thass-Thienemann 1968). The temperature, dryness, moisture, firmness, and smoothness of the skin reveals the quality of the plasma tissue (Pole 2006).

There are many symbolic meanings and somatic metaphors that relate to the skin. Such as, 'you get under my skin', 'to save one's skin', or 'to jump out of one's skin'. The reactions of the skin are an integral expression of what is happening throughout and within the body. Skin reacts to various emotions and has an expressive language of its own.

Table 9.7 Teeth

Glands — Anterior pituitary	Parathyroid	Thyroid	Thymus	Posterior pituitary	Intermediate lobe of pituitary	Pineal	Pineal	Pineal	Pineal	Intermediate lobe of pituitary	Posterior pituitary	Thymus	Thyroid	Parathyroid	Anterior pituitary
Organs — Heart, Small intestine, Endocrine gland, Pericardial	Right breast, Thyroid, Stomach, Pancreas	Lungs, Large intestine	Lungs, Large intestine		Liver, Gallbladder, Eye			Kidneys, Prostate, Bladder, Uterus, Rectum, Anus		Liver, Gallbladder, Eye		Lungs, Large intestine	Lungs, Large intestine	Esophagus, left breast, Thyroid, Stomach, Spleen	Heart, Small intestine, Endocrine gland, Pericardial
Teeth / Upper jaw — 1 3rd molar (wisdom)	2 2nd molar	3 1st molar	4 2nd bicuspid (pre-molar)	5 1st bicuspid (pre-molar)	6 Canine (cuspid)	7 Lateral Incisor	8 Central Incisor	9 Central incisor	10 Lateral Incisor	11 Canine (cuspid)	12 1st bicuspid (pre-molar)	13 2nd bicuspid (pre-molar)	14 1st molar	15 2nd molar	16 3rd molar (wisdom)
Teeth / Lower jaw — 3rd molar (wisdom)	2nd molar	1st molar	2nd bicuspid (pre-molar)	1st bicuspid (pre-molar)	Canine (cuspid)	Lateral Incisor	Central Incisor	Central incisor	Lateral Incisor	Canine (cuspid)	1st bicuspid (pre-molar)	2nd bicuspid (pre-molar)	1st molar	2nd molar	3rd molar (wisdom)
Teeth — 32	31	30	29	28	27	26	25	24	23	22	21	20	19	18	17
Organs — Heart, Small intestine, Endocrine gland, Pericardial	Lungs	Large intestine	Pancreas	Stomach	Liver, Eye			Kidneys, Prostate, Bladder, Uterus, Rectum, Anus		Liver, Eye	Stomach, Spleen		Large intestine	Lungs	Heart, Small intestine, Endocrine gland, Pericardial
Glands — Testicles	Right breast, ovaries				Testicles	Adrenals		Ovaries	Adrenals	Testicles					Testicles, left breast

Source: http://raveecoholistic.com

The blushing of the cheeks, though it seems to be merely a reflex, is the language of the skin expressive of shame, modesty, or embarrassment. In the same way paling is expressive of an 'appalling' effect; 'goose flesh' is also an automatic reaction independent of conscious control, yet expressive of special qualities of fear (Thass-Thienemann 1968).

The condition of the skin reflects the condition of the interior, and the internal condition is either causing or caused by the external condition. Without the surface, there is no inside, and without the inside, there is no surface. When skin is healthy it has a relatively smooth surface. Various marks appearing on the skin result from abnormal internal conditions (Kushi 1979). These marks are a form of discharge from the internal organs, glands, tissues, and muscles, and are a manifestation of the energies which are working in the internal part of our body.

The assessment of the skin involves observation and palpation of the skin's tone and color, moles, markings, eruptions, elasticity, adherence, as well as sites of inflammation and disease. Discoloration of the skin indicates disharmony in an organ system or a specific quality. For example: yellow is often associated with disorders of the liver and gallbladder (fire), red is associated with excesses in the circulatory system (air) or excess of heat, pale is associated with disorders in the respiratory system (air) and also with an overall deficiency state or cold, dark is associated with disorders in the elimination of the kidneys (earth), purple is associated with respiratory and circulatory system (air), and milky white is associated with imbalances in the lymphatic system (water) or a build up of mucus (water). The following indicates how the qualities of the five elements are conveyed on the skin:

- *Air.* Excess results in dry, cold, rough and chapped skin with cracks on hands and feet. Skin concerns often appear in variable areas of the skin. Skin is often dull, dark, and lacking in luster.
- *Fire.* Excess results in symptoms that are red and hot; deficiency results in pallor. A patient with a fire constitution is more prone to rashes and acne and their skin is often freckled or might have moles.
- *Water.* Excess results in plumb and oily skin; deficiency results in dryness. Patients with a water constitution often have smooth, oily skin with a smooth texture.
- *Earth.* Excess increases in thickness; deficiency results in thinness and loss of structure. Patients with an earth constitution have thicker skin that has a tendency to be tough and drier.

FINGERS AND TOES

The hands and feet display the patterns of every part of the body. There are four fingers and a thumb and five toes and each digit has five components; each one representing a part of the body (Lad 2006) (refer to Fig. 9.11, Table 9.8). The foot has two main functions: to support the body's weight and to seamlessly transfer that weight onto a variety of surfaces with each step.

Physical assessment

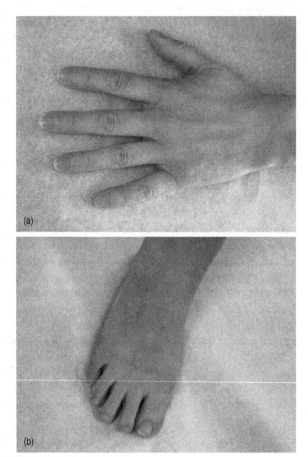

Fig 9.11 Fingers and toes. See Table 9.8.

Fingers represent acute patterns; toes represent chronic or long-standing patterns. A foot is the

> most elaborate structure in the human body and is made up of twenty-eight bones, thirty-three joints, one-hundred and seven ligaments, thirty-one tendons, and miles of nerves and blood vessels. Half of all bones in your body are in the feet (Mogul 2002).

The hands and feet are the most distal parts of the body. Energy flows from the center of the body to the periphery and then returns back to the center. As

Table 9.8 Fingers and toes (Lloyd 2005)		
Element	*Fingers/toes*	*Digits*
Ether	Thumb/big toe	Distal portion (farthest away)
Air	1st finger/toe	Distal joint
Fire	2nd finger/toe	Middle portion
Water	ring finger/toe	Proximal joint
Earth	baby finger/toe	Proximal portion (closest to the body)

the movement throughout the body becomes blocked, it causes constrictions and alters the look of the hands and the feet. For example, you can see tension in a body by observing toes that are bent, raised or gripping the ground. The tension in the toes corresponds to tension in the muscles, either in the neck, back, hips, or the legs, or all of the above.

Guidelines for assessing the fingers and toes

The following are some additional general guidelines:

Assess fingers and toes when they are relaxed. To assess the fingers, have your patient shake their hands and drop them on a flat surface. This way you see how the fingers land in their natural state. If you tell a patient you are going to assess their hands and ask them to place them on a surface they are more likely to compensate by straightening out their hands or equally spacing the fingers.

Follow a similar process when assessing the toes. Ask patients to just relax their feet. Observe a patient's toes when they are sitting on a chair to minimize the impact of gravity, then have them stand up and see if patterns change when they are 'carrying the full weight of their body'.

- Notice what pattern stands out the most on the first glance.
- The fingers and toes are part of a dynamic system, they are constantly changing. Remember that you are looking at a point in time – the pattern might be unwinding or might be just settling in.
- Any pattern can start from internal (thoughts or emotions) or from external (poor shoes); the end result is the same.
- There is normally equal spacing between all the fingers.
- Toes are normally in immediate contact with each other (equal spacing).
- When assessing the hands look for how raised or flat the overall hand is. This indicates how grounded a patient is currently.
- When assessing the feet look at the distribution of weight on the foot. This indicates an internal or external pattern.
- The top portion of the toes represents what a patient shows the world; the energy that manifests outwardly; The bottom portion of the toes, the part that rests on the ground, represents the internal qualities of that component.

When assessing the feet there are many different aspects, each which conveys part of the pattern. The aspects include: alignment, color, lines/marking, spacing, size and shape. Fig. 9.12 illustrates how alignment and spacing are revealed.

Alignment

- *Raised portion* refers to a toe that does not sit flat on the ground. It indicates daydreaming, imagination, lack of being grounded, or a chronic illness (constricted pattern). The degree of the digit that is raised indicates the aspect of the element that is ungrounded.
- *Lateral deviation* is movement either away from the core, towards the external, or towards the future. It can be due to spending more energy in external activities or on being influenced by your external environment more so than your own or focusing more on the present.
- *Medial deviation* indicates movement toward the core, away from the external, or focusing on the past. It can be due to excessive meditation or

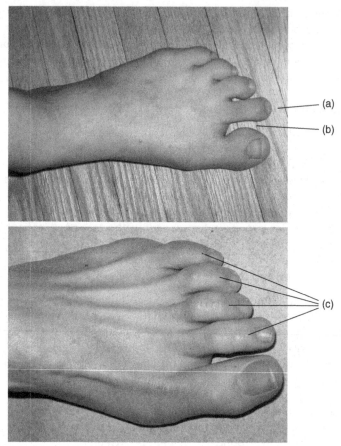

Fig 9.12 Alignment and spacing of toes (a) Long air toe – tendency for the mind to be overactive; (b) large space between ether and air toes – indicates that the person needs time to integrate information; (c) bent toes – sign of constriction or tension in the body.

inward focus, dwelling on the past or avoiding and pulling away from the future or external influences.

- *Twist/tilt* indicates that an individual is showing the world something different than what they feel or think. Where the twist or tilt starts tells you what element is out of balance in its expression. Often it indicates a path that is not straight within an element's expression. For example, a twisted earth toe can reflect issues with elimination or can indicate that someone has issues with how they look.
- *Gripping* indicates fear, shyness, or very sensitive nature with respect to an element. Often there is a sense of constriction and protection of expression. For example, when a patient has a lot of fears their toes will tend to grip the earth.

Color

- *Increased color* indicates increased energy in an element, tension or congestion. Grays and browns reflect crystallized energy that remains to be cleared. Red and pink reflect current issues that are being addressed/shown. The darker the color, the more crystallized the energy. Dark means an excess of heat or cold depending on the rest of the pattern.

- *Decrease in color* indicates decreased energy in an element, weakened or lack of energetic flow. Constriction of blood vessels is associated with excess cold, Yin state, or energy pulled inward.

Lines/markings

- *Horizontal lines* follow the air current and indicate stressful events or situations that have stressed the mind and body, especially air organs.
- *Vertical lines* follow the water current and indicate metabolic disorders. The digits and placement of the lines provide insight into the element(s) involved and the timing of the events.
- *Markings* indicate areas of constriction or trauma that had a significant impact on the body.

Spacing

- *Wide spaces or gaps* indicate that the length of time for movement between the particular elements is long; the bigger the gap, the more time that is needed for the flow of energy between the elements. For example, if there is a wide space between the ether and the air toe then it indicates that the patient needs time before he/she implements new ideas or changes. If there is a wide gap between the fire and air toe it would indicate that a patient would spend a lot of time thinking about an event before they allowed themselves to feel the emotional impact that it had on them.
- *Narrow space* indicates tight connection between the elements. For example, when all the toes are close together a patient would react and process information quickly.
- *Overlapping* indicates that one element is covering for the other, or that the expression of the underlying element is being overshadowed by the element literally on top. For example, if the water toe is hidden under the fire toe it indicates that the patient nurtures himself or herself when emotional. This might show up as eating emotionally or going shopping when upset. If the air toe is on top of the fire toe it indicates that a patient intellectualizes their emotions. They will have a tendency to jump to the logical reason why something is the way it is, often without realizing the emotional impact it has on them.

Size

- *Long* indicates that the particular element is one of prominence for the individual. If the length is out of proportion to the other elements it indicates an area where there is a lot of activity or where the patient spends too much time and finds it difficult to move smoothly to the other elements. If all the toes are long it indicates that a patient can handle a lot of energetic input from many different sources. These people tend to be comfortable and tend to fit into in a variety of different situations.

- *Short* indicates that the particular element is lacking for the individual or it is not an element of prominence. It also indicates directness and spontaneity or the ability of a thought/emotion to move through that element quickly. It is important to look for the specific aspects of a digit that are out of proportion (e.g. short fire aspect of the water toe). For example, if the big toe is short relative to the other toes, it indicates that the patient is easily put into chaos as the energies flow into ether (there isn't enough space (ether) to absorb all the other energies).
- *Wide* indicates a fullness to an element, its strength and openness of expression.
- *Narrow* indicates a constriction to an element, lack of development, or lack of expression.

Shape

- *Rounded edge* indicates someone who is tactful in his or her expression, soft and gentle.
- *Blunt edge* indicates someone who says it like it is and is straightforward, honest, and blunt.
- *Pointy edge* indicates someone who has a tendency to let things build up and then expresses things sharply with direction and force.
- *Bunion* is caused by a large lateral shift of the ether toe. It reflects a pull from the external environment away from the core.
- *Lump* indicates that the expression of a quality of the element is blocked and will be obscured. The placement of the lump reveals the pattern. For example, a lump on the air joint of the fire toe reveals a blockage of emotions (fire toe) in an air aspect of the body (i.e., the lung or nervous system).
- *Fullness on the underside of a toe* indicates that aspects of expression of the element are hid from view of the observer or not expressed fully. For example, if there is a lot of thickness under the right air toe it reveals that there is a lot of mental activity or intellect that the patient has that they don't express or reveal to others.
- *Bottleneck* is the area that is compressed. It indicates where that element gets stuck, is blocked or has difficulty being expressed.
- *Raised bends* occur at the joints and indicate a lack of groundedness, constriction or tension in either the air or water elements. The most distal joint is the air joint and the most proximal joint is the water joint. For example, in arthritis it is common to see the water joint on all toes swollen and raised.
- *Depressed bend* indicates weakness or exhaustion in a particular aspect of a joint.

The following is a sample of how the physical exam and the holistic intake are integrated.

Case 9.1

A 38-year-old female, who is a schoolteacher, is recently separated and lives on her own. Chief complaints are abdominal pain when she eats fatty food, spotting in the middle of her period and some weakness in left knee when she exercises.

What you notice first.	High intense energy level.	Excess pattern
How she looks	Muscular, moderate build with fine features	Fire build. Not a lot of earth
Speech patterns	Rapid, sharp, not a lot of details, impatient	Excess fire, presence of air or a reflection of a deficiency of earth
Change in affect	(a) Talk about paying bills increases the intensity of her voice and it becomes broken (b) Voice slows down when she talks of recent separation and she diverts her eyes. The separation was a surprise to her	(a) Deficiency of internal earth with a lack of water (flow) (b) Deficiency of internal water (nurturing). It could also represent a deficiency in earth if she interprets the separation as not trusting herself
Key words/ phrases	(a) Concern about paying bills (b) Frustrated because she is single (c) She's getting too old to have children	(a) Lack of internal earth (b) Excess fire because of a deficiency in water (relationships) (c) A water concern
Lifestyle energy	(a) Busy at school. Likes her job (b) Good relationship with family (c) High impact exercises for about 2 hours a day. (d) Not eating on a regular basis because she doesn't enjoy cooking for one person	(a) Fire with strong external water (b) Strong external water (c) Excess fire (d) Deficiency of water
Psychological	Usually optimistic Concerned that her health is starting to change in a way that she can't get a handle on and a concern that she is running out of time	Positive Lack of earth and a fire imbalance
Questionnaire	(a) History of broken left ulnar bone 5 years ago (b) Digestive concerns as a teenager (c) Fear and a feeling of not belonging when her parents divorced at 12 years old	(a) Deficiency of earth (b) Susceptibility in a fire system. Fire held internally and not expressed (c) Earth emotions due to a disruption in water (relationships)
Walking	Quick, slight favoring of the right side	Fire with a Yang pattern

(Continued)

Case 9.1—Cont'd

Structural	Full ROM in upper body and spine. Decreased extension of left knee	Deficiency of earth (knee is the negative pole of earth) with a Yin weakness and excess of air (worry) about moving forward in life
	Right hand more forward Left side more contracted from the shoulder to the hip	Yang excess pattern
Functional		
Tongue diagnosis	Red, especially on the sides, thick white coat in the center and scalloping on the sides	Fire with a deficiency of internal water (not digesting and absorbing food)
Pulse diagnosis	Rapid overall, liver pulse is tight	Fire
Chief concerns (CC)	CCI – digestive pain when eats fatty foods CCII – spotting in the middle of her period CCIII – weakness of the left knee	CCI – deficiency of fire CCII – deficiency of earth in the reproductive system (water) CCIII – deficiency of earth (knee is the negative pole of earth) and excess of air (worry) about moving forward in life

REFERENCES

Bar M, Tootell R, Schacter DL, et al 2001 Cortical mechanisms of explicit visual object recognition. Neuron 29:529–535

Baron-Cohen S, Wheelwright S, Jolliffe T 1997 Is there a 'language of the eyes'? Evidence from normal adults, and adults with autism or Asperger syndrome. Visual Cognition 4(3):311–331

Biederman I 1987 Recognition by components: A theory of human image understanding. Psychol Rev 94:115–147

Bridges L 2004 Face Reading in Chinese Medicine. Churchill Livingstone, Missouri

Chaitow L 1997 Palpation Skills, Assessment and Diagnosis through Touch. Churchill Livingstone, New York

Hahnemann S 1997 Organon of Medicine, sixth edition. B. Jain Publishers, New Delhi

Hammer LI 2005 Chinese Pulse Diagnosis, a Contemporary Approach, revised edition. Eastland Press, Seattle

Hanawalt N 1994 The role of the upper and lower parts of the face as the basis for judging facial expressions: II. In posed expressions and 'candid camera' pictures. J Gen Psychol 31:23–36

Hardie S, Hancock P, Rodway P, Penton-Voak I, Carson D, Wright L 2005 The enigma of facial asymmetry: Is there a gender-specific pattern of facedness? Laterality 10(4): 295–304

Jones PB 1991 How to Improve your Eyesight Without Using Glasses or Contact Lenses. Four Winds Publishing, Canada

Kuriyama S 1999 The Expressiveness of the Body and the Divergence of Greek and Chinese Medicine. Zone Books, New York

Kushi M 1983 Your Face Never Lies. Avery Publishing, New Jersey

Lad V 1998 Ayurvedic, the Science of Self-healing. Motilal Banarsidass, Delhi

Lad V 2006 Textbook of Ayurveda, a Complete Guide to Clinical Assessment. Vol 2. The Ayurvedic Press, New Mexico

Liggett J 1974 The Human Face. Stein & Day, New York

Lloyd I 2005 Messages from the Body, a Guide to the Energetics of Health. Naturopathic Foundations, Ontario

Maciocia G 1989 The Foundation of Chinese Medicine. Churchill Livingstone, Edinburgh

Maciocia G 1998 The Foundations of Chinese Medicine. Churchill Livingstone, Edinburgh

Mason MF, Cloutier J, Macrae CN 2006 On constructing others: category and stereotype activation from facial cues. Social Cognition 24(5):540–562

Mattsson B, Mattsson M 2002 The concept of 'psychosomatic' in general practice. Reflections on body language and a tentative model for understanding. Scand J Prim Health Care, 20:135–138

Mogul S 2002 Perfect Feet, Caring and Pampering. Stewart, Tabori & Chang, New York

Nummenmaa T 1964 The Language of the Face. Jyvaskyla, Finland

Ohashi W 1991 Reading the Body, Ohashi book of Oriental Diagnosis. Penguin Group, New York

Oshman J 2003 Energy Medicine in Therapeutics and Human Performance. Butterworth-Heinemann, Edinburgh

Pole S 2006 Ayurvedic Medicine, the Principles of Traditional Practice. Elsevier, Philadelphia

Thass-Thienemann T 1968 Symbolic Behavior. Washington Square Press, New York

Zhen LS 1985 Pulse Diagnosis. Paradigm Publications, Massachusetts

FURTHER READING

Baron RJ 1985 An introduction to medical phenomenology: I can't hear you while I'm listening. Ann Intern Med 103:606–611

González-Crussi F 2007 A Short History of Medicine. Random House, New York

Graves R, Goodglass H, Landis T 1982 Mouth asymmetry during spontaneous speech. Neuropsychologia 20:371–381

Hausmann M, Behrendt-Körbitz S, Kautz H, Lamm C, Radelt F, Gunturkun O 1998 Sex differences in oral asymmetries during word repetition. Neuropsychologia 36(12):1397–1402

Hilarion 1982 Body Signs, the Hidden Meaning of the Foot, Leg, Internal Organs, Vertebra. Marcus Books, Ontario

Lindlahr H 1985 Iridiagnosis and other diagnostic methods, Natural Therapeutics Vol. 4. Hillman Printers, England

Loring DW, Meador KJ, Allison JD, Wright JC 2000 Relationship between motor and language activation using fMRI. Neurology 54:981–983

Marr D 1982 Vision. Freeman, San Francisco

Posner MI, Keele SW 1968 On the genesis of abstract ideas. J Exp Psychol 77:353–363

Reiser SJ 1978 Medicine and the Reign of Technology. Cambridge University Press, England

Rosch E et al 1976 Basic objects in natural categories. Cogn Psychol 8:382–439

Sills F 1989 The Polarity Process, energy as a healing art. Element, Dorset

Somogi I 1997 Reading Toes, Your Feet as Reflections of Your Personality. CW Daniel Company, UK

Svoboda RE 1989 Prakruti, your Ayurvedic Constitution. Geocom, New Mexico

Tao L 1989 How to Read Faces. Hamlyn Publishing Group, London

The Yellow Emperor's Classic of Internal Medicine 1972 University of California Press, Berkeley. In González-Crussi F 2007 A Short History of Medicine. Random House, New York

Voyer D 1996 On the magnitude of laterality effects and sex differences in functional literalities. Laterality 1:51–83

CHAPTER 10
Disease patterns

Often when a patient comes to see a naturopathic practitioner they have already been diagnosed with a disease. Every disease, and its associated symptoms, carries a pattern that assists the practitioner in determining the causal factors. A practitioner's knowledge of the pathophysiology and the etiology of disease assists in guiding the breadth of the holistic intake, physical exam, and associated tests. For example, if a patient presents with cholelithiasis during the intake a practitioner would be listening and looking for factors that are associated with gallbladder concerns, such as dyspepsia, intolerance to fatty foods, belching, bloating, fullness, and nausea (Merck Manual 1999). As the gallbladder is a fire organ (see Table 5.6) a practitioner would also be listening and looking for lifestyle and external factors that have a 'fire' quality, such as increased alcohol consumption, spicy hot food; situations that are irritating, frustrating, or that cause anger; cigarettes or medications that 'heat' up the body; and a life style that a patient feels is too hectic or too busy.

Every disease conveys a pattern with specific qualities and attributes. Together they tell a story and reveal a pattern of disharmony. This pattern relates back to the disrupting factors. When exploring the qualities and characteristics of diseases it is important to remember that there can be more than one explanation for any symptom. For example, a lack of water, an excess of fire, and an excess of air all cause dryness; stiffness can be due to an excess of earth or a lack of water. Human beings are dynamic, complex systems with all parts networked in a specific pattern. The factors behind disease are multi-factorial and the site of disease does always indicate where the disease pattern originated. When assessing a disease, look for the range of possibilities and the relationship between all parts of the body.

STEPS TO THE ASSESSMENT OF DISEASE PATTERNS

The aim of assessing the patterns of disease is to see how the qualities and characteristics of a patient's diseases and symptoms overlap with the qualities and characteristics of the patient's temperament, lifestyle, life events, and external factors. The following steps provide a guide for determining the patterns of diseases.

Level of manifestation

Start by identifying the organ system, or part of the body that is associated with the primary and secondary levels of manifestation. All systems of the body are networked, as well as all levels of the body, and within each network there is a hierarchical relationship between the parts. Identifying the primary and secondary levels of manifestation provides a guide as to the relationship between the levels. For example, if the chief concern is chronic neck pain the practitioner would want to assess the whole structural aspect of the body due to the relationship and correlation between the neck and other structural parts of the body. Likewise, the assessment would also include functional and psychological causes of neck pain. The following are examples of the level of manifestation of different parts of the body:

- scoliosis – structural is primary, psychological and functional are secondary

- dysmenorrhea – functional is primary, psychological and structural are secondary
- anxiety – psychological is primary, functional and structural are secondary.

Element of organ or system

Identify the organ or system associated with the primary level and the element associated with that organ or system. This provides the overall pattern or area of disharmony, the characteristics then provide the specifics. Refer to tables in Chapter 5 to determine the elemental correlation of the organs and systems. For example:

- nervous and respiratory system are a characteristic of the air element
- muscles and digestive system are a characteristic of the fire element
- lymphatic and reproductive systems are a characteristic of the water element
- urinary system and bones are a manifestation of the earth element.

Characteristics of symptom patterns

Identify the signs and symptoms that are being manifested, and the associated qualities and characteristics. Identify the characteristics associated with both the primary and the secondary levels of manifestation. For example, if the chief concern was asthma the characteristics associated with the respiratory system (primary level) would be considered as well as those associated with the psychological and structural levels, which are secondary. The symptoms that manifest indicate the stage and progression of disease.

Chapter 5 explores symptom patterns in detail, such as the patterns of internal and external, Yin–Yang, excess and deficiency, and the five elements. There is often a blending of the qualities, such as an excess of fire, a deficiency of Yang. The symptom pattern can either mirror or balance the disrupting factor. For example, if the disrupting factor is the consumption of too much food that is causing dampness, the symptom will likely be one of dampness, if the disrupting factor involves worrying too much (excess air) the body may balance that disruption with a symptom of constricted or deficiency of air, i.e., wheezing in the lungs, or constipation. Below is a review of the five elements and a look at how excesses and deficiencies in these elements might manifest.

- *Earth* represents the strength and structure of the organs. An excess of earth is seen as a decrease in flexibility, stiffness, and heaviness. The formation of cysts, tumors, or lumps denotes an earth quality. Earth conditions also tend to be more consistent and deep. A deficiency of earth is seen as an inability of body parts to hold their structure or shape or to keep things in. A deficiency of earth also manifests as weakness or atrophy.
- *Water* is the fluid aspect of the body and relates to the production of body fluids. Swelling and an increase in weight or the presence of fluid are signs of excess water. Dehydration and dryness are signs of deficiency. A deficiency of water manifests as areas feeling cold and weak or empty, or a lack of body fluids.

- *Fire* is the impulse behind movement. It denotes the warmth of the body. Excess fire is seen when areas are red and hot. Irritability, frustration, and restlessness are also signs of excess fire. A deficiency of fire manifests as a lack of enthusiasm or motivation, a lack of impulse to move, or a lack of warmth.
- *Air* is the primary element of movement especially as it relates to the nervous system. Air imbalances are seen as pain that moves around, symptoms that come and go at random, and/or the presence of gas, and dryness.
- *Ether* is represented by the quality of space. An ether imbalance occurs when there is the sense of not having enough space, or not liking the space you're in.

Nature of signs and symptoms

The nature of signs and symptoms provides information on the onset, intensity, and frequency of the symptoms (refer to Chapter 6). It also provides information on the degree that the symptom pattern has impacted health. The nature of signs and symptoms provides an insight as to the factors that have disrupted health and the length of time an individual has been in a state of overwhelm.

Associated signs and symptoms

Symptoms are considered associated with each other when they relate to the same organ or system, or when the onset started around the same time. Symptoms that are associated by timing or the same triggers are often part of the same pattern. Associated signs and symptoms can also be an indication of the progressive nature of a disease pattern. Each associated sign and symptom can be further assessed using the same criteria described above. In doing so, the window of assessment often becomes more focused on deeper subsystems of the human network. The same principles of assessment apply. For the purpose of the examples below the associated signs and symptoms will not be included.

Aggravating and ameliorating factors

The awareness of aggravating and ameliorating factors assists a practitioner in clarifying the causal factors and the patterns of systems and diseases. This awareness is captured in the holistic intake.

Cause of disruption

This last step involves relating the patterns of disease to a patient's temperament, lifestyle, life events, or environmental and external factors. It involves relating the patient's subjective recall of their life to the practitioner's objective findings. Once the pattern of the symptoms and disease has been assessed, and the factors that have contributed to the disruption have been identified, a treatment strategy can be determined.

Rheumatoid arthritis (RA)

RA is defined as a chronic syndrome characterized by non-specific, usually symmetric inflammation of the peripheral joints, potentially resulting in progressive destruction of articular and periarticular structures (Merck Manual 1999).

- *Level of manifestation.* Arthritis primarily affects the structural aspect of the body, with the functional and psychological being secondary.
- *Element of organ or system.* Joints are associated with the ether element and they relate to the relative freedom of movement of the body. Joints allow for movement, the extent of which is determined by their structure and alignment (Legge 1997).
- *Characteristics of symptom pattern*

  - *Inflammation and swelling* – excess of water, the presence of redness and heat brings in the fire quality as well. Determine if the swelling is localized to the synovial membrane or spread to the ligaments, tendons, tendon sheath and bursa; if it has it indicates a progressive worsening of the disease. Inflammation and swelling is associated with an increased ESR reading.
  - *Anemia* is a sign of a decrease in internal earth.
  - *Pain and stiffness which is worse after rest* – an earth imbalance or a lack of water (flow).
  - *Weakness and lethargy* – a deficiency of earth or a decrease in overall vitality.
  - *Subcutaneous nodules* – an earth imbalance, often due to a lack of flow.
  - *Destruction of articular and periarticular structures* – a deficiency of earth.
  - *Peripheral joints* are an external feature. The periphery relates to a patient's relationship with the external. RA usually affects the small joints first then spreads symmetrically and centripetally, indicating a Yin pattern is affecting a greater aspect of the person's life.
  - *RA factor* denotes an autoimmune component which indicates a deeper pathology and a disconnect between a person's life and their personal essence, or sense of self (an earth – ether imbalance).
  - *Specific fingers or joints* – if RA involves specific fingers or joints, look at the qualities of the specific areas that are affected. For example, it is common for all the water joints (proximal interphalangeal joints) on the hands to be affected. If RA is worse on either the right or left this provides insight into a Yin–Yang pattern.

Nature of signs and symptoms

'The onset of RA is usually insidious, with progressive joint involvement, but may be abrupt, with simultaneous inflammation in multiple joints' (Merck Manual 1999). A gradual onset is often associated with ongoing lifestyle, social, or environmental factors. When the onset is abrupt, look for a situation or event that triggered an immediate state of overwhelm. RA can be transient, gradual, or progressive. RA is more likely to be transient when there is an external situation that contributes to the imbalance that resolves. If the situation doesn't resolve, the progression is more likely to be gradual. Excesses and deficiencies in the building blocks to health aggravate, flare up RA, and add to the progressive nature.

RA pattern

Overall, RA is an ether imbalance due to disharmony between what a patient desires in their life and what they are doing; or an imbalance between what is beneficial for a patient and their lifestyle. It manifests as a deficiency of earth (structural changes in the joint or decrease in circulation to the joint) and an imbalance of water (swelling). Look for areas in a person's life that are restrictive or a lifestyle that is too structured or controlled, with a lack of nurturing, creativity, or enjoyment. Also address those lifestyle factors that are not aligned to a patient's constitution.

Osteoporosis

Osteoporosis is defined as a generalized progressive diminution of bone density, causing skeletal weakness. The net rate of bone resorption exceeds the rate of bone formation, resulting in a decrease in overall bone mass (Merck Manual 1999).

- *Level of manifestation.* The structural level is primary, the functional and psychological are secondary.
- *Element of organ or system.* Bone is a quality of the earth element.
- *Characteristics of symptom pattern*

  - *Often asymptomatic*, especially in the early stages which indicates that the causal factors are more likely to be due to disruptions in the secondary sites.
  - *Pain* can occur in the bone or muscle especially if the osteoporosis is in the spine, if the pain is localized look at the patterns relating to that particular spot, or the structure of that part of the body. Overall pain is an air attribute. With osteoporosis the pain is often dull and localized indicating more of an earth pattern.
  - *Weakness* is a deficiency symptom.
  - *Sidedness.* Osteoporosis can occur anywhere in the body. Often, there is a difference right to left indicating a Yin–Yang pattern; a difference in the hip versus the spine might indicate a difference between someone's core strength and the support they have for moving forward with their life or the support they feel from others.
  - *Decrease in calcium and other minerals, as well as a decrease in the organic matrix of bone* – a deficiency of earth (minerals) and water (nutrients).

Nature of signs and symptoms

Typically osteoporosis has a gradual onset, indicating more of a lifestyle pattern or the influence of external factors. If the bone density of a patient shows a dramatic change in a short period of time, look for situations or life events that significantly affected them.

Osteoporosis pattern

Osteoporosis is a deficiency of internal earth. It is a result of the accumulation of factors that build earth and those that weaken earth. The factors that build earth include: a diet that is high in minerals (root vegetables and greens), strong posture and physical alignment, ongoing exercise and movement, and a sense of feeling strong, safe, secure, supported, and protected. Factors that weaken earth include: feeling fearful, vulnerable, and unsure, a poor diet and one that is acid, poor posture, etc. The patterns of Yin and Yang, external and internal, come into play depending on the bones that are deficient. For some people, the primary contributing factor is an internal deficiency of earth (lack of internal strength or feeling supported); for others it is primarily due to external factors; such as lifestyle, diet, sleep; exercise. Calcium, the primary mineral in bone, is used to balance acidity in the blood. Acidity is often due to excesses in a patient's life, such as coffee, soft drinks, or high protein diets. The deficiency in the bones may be balancing the excesses in lifestyle.

Acute bronchitis

Bronchitis is defined as acute inflammation of the tracheobronchial tree, generally self-limiting, and with eventual complete healing and return of function (Merck Manual 1999). Bronchitis is typically a result of a weakened immune system that is overwhelmed by exposure to an external factor, such as bacteria or viruses, or air pollution. From a naturopathic perspective, the focus would include the increased susceptibility of the patient. A weakened immune system results from factors that negatively affect digestive function, such as improper dietary habits, poor food choices, excesses or deficiencies in diet, and food intolerances; or factors that negatively affect respiratory function, such as a sedentary lifestyle, inhaled pollutants and toxins, or improper breathing. The immune system can also be weakened by psychological and structural factors.

- *Level of manifestation.* The functional level is primary, the psychological and structural are secondary.
- *Element of organ or system.* The lungs are associated with the air element.
- *Characteristics of symptom pattern.* The symptoms associated with acute bronchitis indicate an acute healing response and include:

  o *Inflammation* – a water and fire pattern.
  o *Wheezing, or bronchial constriction* – a decrease in air (movement) and an excess in earth (constriction)
  o *Phlegm* – a water and earth imbalance. The more yellow the phlegm, the more the influence of the quality of fire (bacteria).
  o *Sidedness* – if congestion in the lungs is more right or left sided, this provides a Yin–Yang quality. The sidedness is determined by auscultation and by palpation.

Nature of signs and symptoms

The frequency of the bronchitis attacks indicates the level of susceptibility in the lung. It also relates to the frequency of triggers and the strength of the internal body. Bronchitis is usually self-limiting and mild. This relates to situations where the imbalance in a person's life is temporary. If a patient suffers from bronchitis repeatedly it indicates that the lungs or the air element are areas of susceptibility, it can also indicate that previous bronchitis episodes were suppressed.

Pattern of acute bronchitis

Overall, acute bronchitis represents disharmony between the internal and the external. It is due to an imbalance in the air element, an internal deficiency of water and earth, and an external excess focus. In other words, a patient who focused a lot on other people, projects, or responsibilities (external excess), and does not take care of themselves (internal deficiency). The most susceptible person is someone who has a weakened immune system (deficiency of internal earth), is malnourished (internal deficiency pattern) or who thinks or worries (excess air) that it is more important to nurture and take care of others versus themselves (water imbalance) and therefore becomes exhausted and weakened (deficiency of earth).

Essential hypertension

Hypertension is defined as an elevation of systolic and/or diastolic blood pressure, either primary or secondary (Merck Manual 1999).

- *Level of manifestation.* The functional level is primary, the psychological and structural are secondary.
- *Element of organ or system.* The circulatory system is a quality of the air element, and blood is a quality of earth. Hypertension refers to the movement of blood throughout the body being constricted.
- *Characteristics of symptom pattern* in many cases,
  - *Asymptomatic* which means that a practitioner needs to look at the associated signs and symptoms to determine the causal factors.
  - *Fire* hypertension is often due to emotions that increase internal heat, such as irritability, frustration, and anger. The more these emotions are held in the body, the greater their impact. Held emotions result in increased constriction of muscles.
  - *Water* hypertension is associated with increased viscosity of the blood and other concerns due to improper kidney function. The increased viscosity is often due to decreased digestive fire and the absorption of undigested food or toxins from the digestive tract. It is also associated with obesity and imbalances in diet or food intolerances.
  - *Earth* hypertension results in stagnation and a break down of tissue and structures. It is associated with earth emotions such as fear and insecurity. It can also relate to build up of cholesterol on the walls of the arteries, which results in an increase in earth and hence increase stiffness.

Nature of associated signs and symptoms

The onset can be either gradual or immediate. A gradual onset is due to lifestyle and external factors. If the onset occurred more suddenly it is often associated with an accident, injury, or trauma – psychological, functional, or structural.

Pattern of hypertension

Hypertension is typically caused by tension or constriction in the blood vessels (excess of fire and earth) or an excess of body fluids (excess water). Improper dietary habits and psychological distress are two common causes for hypertension.

Irritable bowel syndrome (IBS)

IBS is defined as a motility disorder involving the entire gastrointestinal (GI) tract, causing recurring upper and lower GI symptoms, including variable degrees of abdominal pain, constipation and/or diarrhea, and abdominal bloating (Merck Manual 1999).

- *Level of manifestation*. The functional level is primary, the psychological and structural secondary.
- *Element of organ or system*. Digestive system is associated with the fire element. The role of the digestive system is to digest and absorb everything that a person takes in, literally and metaphorically. Metabolism is primarily a fire function, the absorption of nutrients a water function, and the movement throughout the digestive tract is dependant on the nervous system which is an air function. The nervous system is closely linked to thoughts and emotions and to breathing. The digestive system functions optimally in parasympathetic mode. In this mode the body is focused internally. The erratic nature of motility in IBS is associated with the nervous system being in sympathetic mode, or in a state of flight and fight, which is a pattern of external excess.
- *Characteristics of symptom pattern*

  - *Abdominal pain* (hypersensitivity) – an air attribute, yet the pain associated with IBS is typically stabbing, sharp, and intense which are all fire qualities.
  - *Constipation and/or diarrhea* – primarily an air imbalance due to the alternating pattern. See Chapter 5 for a more complete look at pattern of constipation. Water and earth also play a role depending on the nature of the stools.
  - *Abdominal bloating* – an excess of air.
  - *Mucus* production – an excess of earth in the water element.
  - *Anxiety or irritability* – fire emotions, often with excess air as well

Nature of signs and symptoms

Patients diagnosed with IBS often have a history of having GI complaints. This would indicate that the GI system is an organ of susceptibility. This susceptibility may be constitutional, congenital, or due to a lifestyle that is imbalanced for the patient, or due to a situation or event that has never healed appropriately. IBS has an intermittent pattern of systems, which refers to situations or triggers that come and go, such as stressful encounters. More frequent, consistent, and intense symptoms reflect a more continual disrupting factor in a patient's temperament, lifestyle or environment, or a pattern that is more progressed and intense.

Pattern of irritable bowel syndrome

IBS is a fire imbalance due to an external excess of air, and an internal deficiency of water. In other words, when there are situations that bother a patient they are likely to hold in their thoughts and emotions (contracted energy and Yin pattern) in their digestive system (fire). Situations that are irritating, frustrating, that cause anger, or that involve a lack of nurturing or creativity are the most likely triggers. Foods that have quality of excess fire or a deficiency of water might also trigger IBS. IBS is a functional disorder often with no evidence of accompanying structural defects, i.e., the earth is in tack.

Multiple sclerosis (MS)

'A slowly progressive central nervous system (CNS) disease characterized by disseminated patches of demyelination in the brain and spinal cord, resulting in multiple and varied neurologic symptoms and signs, usually with remissions and exacerbations' (Merck Manual 1999). In experiments looking at the light that was emitted around various tissues it was found that MS was in a state of too much order. The patients were taking in too much light and this was inhibiting the cells from doing their job, in other words, MS patients were drowning in light (McTaggart 2002). Whereas with most other diseases, it was found that there was too little order.

- *Level of manifestation.* The functional level is primary, the psychological and the structural are secondary.
- *Element of organ or system.* The nervous system is a characteristic of the air element.
- *Characteristics of symptom pattern*

  - *Plaques of demyelination* – a deficiency of earth.
  - *Perivascular inflammation* – an excess of water and fire.
  - *CNS* – located in the midline or 'core' of a patient representing an internal pattern.
  - *Diffuse neurological signs* – the diffuseness is an air quality, the locations in which the signs and symptoms appear would have their own characteristics and attributes.
  - *Paresthesias* in one or more extremities, in the trunk, or on one side of the face – the nervous system governs all sensations and it is governed by the air element. Paresthesia is a deficiency state due to the lack of consistent sensation and the wandering pattern.
  - *Weakness in a leg or hand* – is a deficiency pattern. The structure and symbolic meaning associated with the parts of the body involved should also be looked at.
  - *Visual disturbances* – vision is governed by the fire element.

Nature of signs and symptoms

The symptoms associated with MS are of *periods of remission and exacerabation* – this is a nature of the air element and it relates to causes that come and go, or to periods of the body being exhausted. It is common for MS symptoms to be worse when a patient is over-extended, lacking sleep, or exhausted.

MS is a progressive disease with the timing and severity of the progression being very individualized. It represents the multifactorial aspect of MS and the uniqueness of each patient.

Pattern of multiple sclerosis

The pattern of MS is an excess of air and a deficiency of earth in the air element. The deficiency of earth occurs in the core (CNS) and relates to a deficiency of internal earth, which can relate to a weakened sense of self, or feeling a lack of support and strength. An excess of air is aggravated by continual mental stimulation, spending a lot time on computers or watching television, a busy hectic lifestyle, and by irregular patterns of sleeping and eating.

REFERENCES

Legge D 1997 Close to the Bone. Sydney College Press, Australia

McTaggart L 2002 The Field, the Quest for the Secret Force of the Universe. HarperCollins, London

Merck Manual Seventeenth Edition. 1999 Merck Research Laboratories, New Jersey

FURTHER READING

Frawley D 1989 Ayurvedic Healing, a Comprehensive Guide. Passage Press, Utah

Lad V 2005 Ayurvedic Perspectives on Selected Pathologies. The Ayurvedic Press, New Mexico

Lloyd IR 2006 Messages from the Body, a Guide to the Energetics of Health. Naturopathic Publications, Toronto

Morningstar A 2001 The Ayurvedic Guide to Polarity Therapy: hands-on healing. Lotus Press, Wisconsin

Pizzorno JE, Murray MT 2000 Textbook of Natural Medicine, second edition. Churchill Livingstone, Edinburgh

Robbins SL et al (eds) 1999 Robbins Pathologic Basis of Disease, sixth edition. WB Saunders Company, Philadelphia

Rossi E 2007 Shen, Psycho-Emotional Aspects of Chinese Medicine. Churchill Livingstone, Philadelphia

Seller RH Differential Diagnosis of Common Complaints, fourth edition. WB Saunders, Philadelphia

Silbernagl S, Lang F 2000 Color Atlas of Pathophysiology. Thiene, Stuttgart

Svoboda RE 1989 Prakuti, your Ayurvedic Constitution. Geocom, New Mexico

SECTION IV
TREATMENT STRATEGIES

CHAPTER 11
Treatment strategies

The intention of naturopathic medicine is to treat the initiating and aggravating factors that are preventing the innate healing ability of the body. It is then to use the most gentle treatments possible to re-establish health and achieve the patient's goals. The naturopathic doctor chooses treatments that restore the natural harmony, rhythm, and coherence to the body. From a conventional medical point of view, treatment is based on the achievement of objective criteria; from a naturopathic medical perspective, treatment is based on achieving the patient's which may be subjective, versus objective goals. From a naturopathic perspective, healing is like cultivating a garden; from a conventional medical perspective it is like fixing a machine.

A practitioner's approach to healing is based on their philosophies and beliefs. Healing, like assessment, is a mindset. The perspective on health, the knowledge of energy patterns and complex systems, the expectations and belief about the purpose of life all influences the healing options and treatment strategy that are chosen, both for a practitioner and a patient. For example, one practitioner might use nutrition and lifestyle counseling, another herbs, another might use acupuncture, another talk therapy, and another hands-on healing. Every practitioner, if they properly assess and treat the causative factors and the pattern of disharmony and if they have a good rapport with a patient, would be able to achieve the same result. The actual healing method does not matter as much as the intention.

A naturopathic treatment plan might involve the use of herbs, supplements, or other treatments, but the focus of treatment involves a shift away from 'what do I take' to 'what do I change.' The role of a practitioner is to facilitate change. They do not 'heal' a patient. It is what the patient does that determines the degree that the body will heal and their ability to maintain a higher level of health. The conventional mode of healing puts the primary focus on the practitioner. The naturopathic approach maintains the focus on the patient. The practitioner has an educative and facilitative role versus a corrective role.

The role of the practitioner is to provide a road map to facilitate the healing process. Healing is work. It requires a patient taking personal responsibility and being willing to change. It requires attention to all aspects of the body, especially those that are displaying patterns of disharmony. A naturopathic doctor balances the need for medical intervention with allowing the healing power of the body to follow its natural course.

The treatment strategy that chosen for a patient depends on the assessment outcomes, as discussed in Chapter 9, the diagnoses, as well as the health goals of the patient, the risk to health, the healing intention, and the patient's constitution, vitality, and will. The aim of this chapter is to highlight the considerations that determine a treatment strategy. Reviewing the range of treatments used in naturopathic medicine is beyond the scope of this book.

SATISFACTORY VERSUS OPTIMAL HEALTH

There is a difference between *satisfactory* health and *optimal* health. Satisfactory health is based on what a patient desires at a specific point in time. For example, a patient might be satisfied if their pain or discomfort is manageable, versus making the necessary changes to ensure that it is completely resolved. Many patients pay attention to their health only when there is a problem, and stop paying attention to it when the immediate concern is alleviated. For many, a healthy lifestyle involves minimizing pain and discomfort, and doing what it takes so that their physical body doesn't interfere with their desired lifestyle.

Satisfactory health often is based on short-term objectives. For example, patients who eat a poor diet and have an unhealthy sedentary lifestyle do so because it is convenient and easy; either because of lack of awareness of the long-term consequences or without regard for the long-term effects. Or a patient who desires to look younger and therefore takes a lot of supplements and medications or does injection therapies. The patient might achieve their short-term ideal health, but in the process they might have impacted their health in the long run. It is not uncommon for patients who desire to lose weight to choose a weight loss scheme that is not healthy and that has nothing to do with addressing the reasons they are carrying excess weight. They might be successful in losing weight initially, but if the underlying cause is not addressed, they often will decrease their overall health and gain the weight back.

Optimal health involves achieving the highest level of health you can in all aspects of your life. It is based on addressing the root causes of symptoms and diseases, living a life that has the building blocks for long-term health, and having a lifestyle that is based on spiritual, mental, emotional, physical, community, and environmental health. Optimal health involves making life decisions with long-term health as the priority. It requires work and attention to all aspects of life and works through health concerns not just suppresses them or gets rid of them. Optimal health relates to the body as a form of two-way communication. As you are able to interpret the message of the body and respond appropriately, you move closer towards optimal health.

Many people live somewhere between searching for satisfactory health and optimal health. The role of the practitioner is to match the treatment plan to the goals of the patient. It is not helpful for a practitioner to offer a treatment that will provide short-term benefits by suppressing the symptoms when the patient is looking for an understanding of the root cause. Likewise, it is not helpful for a practitioner to provide recommendations to a patient to address the root cause when a patient is interested in getting rid of the symptoms. In the latter example, chances are the patient will stop the treatment plan as soon as the symptoms subside.

RISK TO LIFE

To determine the type and treatment strategy that is required, the potential of cure, and the prognosis of any disease, it is helpful to understand the severity of symptoms and the degree to which health and life are at risk. The aim of all treatments is to address the initiating and aggravating factors and to reestablish harmony within the body. How those factors are addressed, the degree of intervention depends on the risk to life and the vitality and healing potential of the individual. Disease exists on the spectrum of mild to incurable.

- *Mild.* When the risk is mild; treatments that address the initiating factor and the building blocks to health and that involve gradual changes often are what are required to restore health.

- *Moderate.* As the progression of disease increases and the disease becomes more chronic, treatment involves lifestyle changes, as well as other supportive therapies. The healing potential of the patient determines the degree to which they are advised to make major changes to their lifestyle and the degree to which they are encouraged to address unresolved issues.
- *High risk* situations arise in two ways: when disease becomes more ingrained in the body and there is degeneration of tissues and organs that are threatening life, and when there is a sudden impact on health. When the risk is high, the aim of treatment is first to save a patient's life. The focus is on alleviating the risk to life, followed by addressing root causes and aggravating factors.
- *Palliative care* is about maximizing quality of life. At this stage, the progression of disease, or the risk to life, is severe and the disease or symptoms are deemed incurable. Palliative care often is associated with the elderly or the end-stage of chronic disease, but it can involve any age group. The aim of treatment is to support the patient, to minimize pain and discomfort, and to provide comfort to the patient.

HEALING INTENTIONS

Intention is the direction, purpose, aim, or goal that we have for doing something (Quinn 1996). Intentions are set both consciously and unconsciously. They are based on a patient's belief system, their expectations and their desire for a specific outcome (McTaggart 2002). The outcome of any treatment depends on the intention of the patient and the practitioner, the depth and accuracy of the assessment, the motivation and ability of the patient to change, the progression of the disease, and the treatments that are used. The intention to 'cure' or 'heal' encompasses the treatment strategies of balance, support, manage, palliate, suppress, or radical intervention.

All modes of treatment cause a shift in health, and they all have their value and purpose. When a patient is bleeding internally because of a ruptured abdominal aorta, initially a radical treatment that focuses on saving their life is more appropriate than one that addresses their deep-seated anger and frustration. The following paragraphs review the different modes of healing. The intention to balance or support health works with the healing power of the body. Treatments that manage, palliate, suppress, or involve a radical intervention might provide the relief that is required for a patient to make the necessary changes in life, but do not directly support the healing power of the body or address the root causes of disease. A patient is able to move from one intention to another. For example they can move from a management strategy, to a supportive and eventually to a balancing strategy if the patient is willing and the healing potential is strong enough.

Balance

Each patient has a unique constitution and susceptibility to certain symptoms and areas of disharmony. On an ongoing basis a patient can choose a lifestyle that balances their susceptibilities and maintains their health.

For example, if a patient has a tendency to be cold and have dry skin, then they would avoid a lot of cold, dry food, especially during the winter. Learning to live in a harmonious way with nature and your constitution involves having a lifestyle that maintains health and balances situations as they are encountered without minimal need for external interventions (Case 11.1).

Case 11.1

A 32-year-old man has a number of mild, intermittent complaints. He has periodic gas and bloating, slight eczema on his elbows, is sometimes tired in the middle of the day, has irregular bowel movements, and is starting to gain weight. During the intake it is found that he has a very hectic job, eats out most of the time, drinks coffee two to three times a day and drinks very little water, stays up late at night working on his computer, and has an irregular exercise schedule. He enjoys his life and has strong relationships with family and friends. He has a fire–earth build and the physical exam reveals forward head posture, shallow breathing, rapid pulse, and a white coat in the center of his tongue. His vital signs are normal and there is nothing remarkable on the blood workup. The treatment strategy involved addressing the building blocks to health, including a diet regimen and food choices that are suited to his constitution, decreasing coffee to one cup in the morning, increasing the consumption of water, education on proper breathing, improving sleeping patterns, and an exercise program that addresses the forward head posture. The symptoms were mild enough that they did not warrant any supplements or supportive therapies. Within a couple of months all the symptoms had resolved. When any of the symptoms periodically returned, he was able to identify the causal factors and to make the necessary changes.

Support

To support means to provide comfort or assistance. Treatments that are supportive assist the body in achieving a higher state of health by providing nutrients, nurture, information, or substances that are required to address a specific symptom or disease. Addressing the building blocks to health, body work, acupuncture, nutrients, botanicals, homeopathy, counseling, etc. can all be used as a form of support to a patient. Supportive treatments decrease the overall burden on the body, they lessen the intensity of the signs and symptoms, and they improve the quality of a patient's life. They involve removing the obstacles to cure and stimulating the inherent healing power of the body. Examples of supportive treatments include: taking specific supplements to remove the buildup of heavy metals in the body and then decreasing ongoing exposure, addressing structural misalignment through hands-on therapy and then modifying posture to prevent its recurrence, modifying diet and taking nutritional supplements to address nutritional deficiencies and intolerances, and using herbs to assist with detoxifying the liver as a patient cuts down on their alcohol use. Many of the treatments used by naturopathic doctors are supportive. These treatments are often used periodically and for a short term with the expectation that when they are completed and the necessary changes in lifestyle and external exposures are made that the body will be able to maintain health on its own by living a life that is in balance with a patient's constitution (Case 11.2).

Case 11.2

A 48-year-old woman presents with anxiety. The anxiety started 3 weeks earlier and is increasing in intensity and frequency. The symptoms associated include shortness of breath, heart palpitations, backache and headache, and nausea. The symptoms started after an incident where she was almost rear-ended on the highway. The patient does have a history of muscle stiffness but has never suffered from anxiety and has found that since it started she is not as comfortable driving. The physical exam revealed fixations of the mid thorax, hypertonicity of neck and lower back muscles, and decreased breathing expansion bilaterally. The initial treatment involved the homeopathic remedy Aconitum 200c (one dose) and a thoracic adjustment. These treatments decreased the anxiety noticeably within 48 hours and the patient was then able to focus on reframing the accident, breathing exercises, and treatments to address the ongoing muscle tension.

Manage

To manage means to control, handle, manipulate, or bring about a desired outcome. Treatments that require the ongoing administration to achieve a specific outcome are in management mode. Many chronic diseases require management, at least initially, for example, diabetes, chronic kidney disease, autoimmune disease, etc. If the progression of disease is advanced, if the patient is advancing in age, or if the goal of the patient is to minimize the symptoms, the treatment intention is to manage.

The intention of management, from a naturopathic perspective, is to provide patients with an increased quality of life and decreased progression of disease. This is accomplished by removing as many causal factors as possible, by considering the interrelationship of all aspects of the patient, and by supporting the body as a unit.

The management of diseases has historically been the focus of conventional treatments. Yet from a conventional medicine perspective, management of symptoms and diseases often includes treatments that produce a desired response in the body irrespective of the other processes that are occurring and the interrelationship among the organs and body systems. Whenever you control solely one aspect of the body it disrupts the ebb and flow of the body as a unit. The improvement in quality of life often is short lived, because other aspects of health are disrupted and start to show signs of imbalance. For example, many patients find themselves taking an increasing number of drugs over time due to the management of signs and symptoms versus the treatment of the underlying triggers or root causes (Case 11.3).

Case 11.3

A 50-year-old man has recently been diagnosed with diabetes and moderate hypertension. He reports that he has been healthy most of his life and enjoys life, which includes fine dining, a good wine, a lot of traveling, and socializing. He does not want the diabetes or hypertension to get worse, but he also doesn't want to dramatically change his life. A treatment strategy in this scenario would involve a lot of education and awareness. Mindfulness exercises and stretching exercises were introduced to decrease the internal constriction and to maintain flexibility. Lifestyle changes included increasing the consumption of water and cutting down on alcohol, removing food intolerances and learning how to choose foods that do not raise the blood sugar. It also involved supplements such as fish oils and herbs to manage the blood pressure and the blood sugar readings to within acceptable ranges. Overtime, the patient incorporated additional lifestyle changes that were beneficial and achieved the goals of managing the diabetes and hypertension; as well as, enjoying life.

Palliate

To palliate means to lessen or ease the pain or discomfort of the symptoms without curing them, to give temporary relief. At times it is necessary to palliate, to remove the intensity of the discomfort, so that a patient has the energy and ability to focus and make necessary changes in their life. Most forms of treatment can be used to palliate. For example, anti-inflammatory herbs to decrease pain, a homeopathic remedy to remove the intensity of anxiety, or body work to lessen the tension in muscles. Palliation can be a valuable treatment strategy in cases such as psychological distress or pain. When used appropriately, and for a short time, palliating symptoms can provide a patient with the relief they require in order to make the necessary changes in their life. If symptoms are palliated repeatedly, or for a long period of time, they will result in a suppression of the symptoms. There is a fine line between palliating and suppressing symptoms. A thorough holistic intake will guide a practitioner as to whether palliation is required (Case 11.4).

Case 11.4

An 80-year-old man is concerned with the constant swelling and discomfort in his legs. He also complains of coldness, shortness of breath, fatigue, and insomnia. His shortness of breath is better as the day goes on. He recently underwent heart surgery and has been previously diagnosed with sleep apnea, hypertension, hypercholesterolemia, and moderate kidney disease. He is on eight different medications for his conditions. Significant blood work findings reveal low reticulocytes, hemoglobin, and leukocytes and decrease glomerular filtration rate (GFR) and increased creatinine. The patient is looking for relief from discomfort, and improvement in sleep. Due to the age of the patient, the progression of disease, and the numerous

Case 11.4—Cont'd

medications, a treatment strategy that involved gradual, gentle changes was advised. The treatment included increasing warming foods, decreasing raw and cold foods, avoiding cold liquids, avoiding foods that cause dampness in the body, and increasing blood-forming foods. He was advised to walk for 5 to 10 minutes before breakfast, and walk 5 minutes every hour. Nutritional supplements were chosen to address the nutritional deficiencies caused by the prescription medication and herbs were prescribed to improve kidney function. Within 2 weeks the swelling and discomfort had dramatically improved and the patient had more energy.

Suppress

To suppress means to subdue, block, dismiss, or to get rid of a symptom without resolving it. Any form of treatment or healing can suppress. Taking drugs to block a rash or to mask any symptom is a form of suppression. Suppressive treatments often provide symptom relief while the underlying disease processes continue unabated. Many drugs work by suppressing symptoms, and the result is that the patient's health progressively deteriorates.

Radical intervention

A radical change is an extreme, often traumatic modification of health. Surgery and drugs, such as chemotherapy, that have an extreme impact on the body, are the most common forms of radical change. What determines the effect of a radical intervention is the connection the patient makes between the event, the outcome, and the intention behind the treatment. If a patient undergoes a life saving heart operation and then dramatically modifies their lifestyle, then the radical intervention is like a 'wake-up call' that will motivate a patient to make the necessary changes to their lifestyle. If, on the other hand, a patient undergoes heart surgery, and sees that as the fix to the problem then they are unlikely to make the changes that are required. Radical interventions are advantageous primarily when the health risks are high.

Case 11.5

A 23-year-old woman presents with a recurrence of Hodgkin lymphoma. The initial sign of recurrence was psoriasis on her thighs and recurring shortness of breath. During the intake the patient noted that she was having difficulties in relationships where she was angry and didn't feel like she could be herself or express her emotions. She reported that her energy had been decreasing over the last month, especially when the recurrence of cancer was confirmed. The physical exam noted decreased breath sounds on the upper right side of the lung, swollen submandibular and clavicular lymph nodes, clubbed nails on all fingers, especially the air finger on the left hand, bare areas were noted on the corresponding lung area of the tongue, and the pulses were deep and weak. The blood pressure was 94/58. Labs reports indicated a mass in the upper right lobe of the lung, lymphadenopathy, and decreased red and white blood cell counts. An ELISA blood test revealed various food intolerances including dairy, corn, wheat, and pineapple. The patient did not feel that she would survive conventional treatment in her current state. For 4 months the patient underwent naturopathic treatments to treat her food intolerances, support her immune, respiratory function, and lymphatic systems, and address the psychological issues. During those 4 months, the patient's blood counts improved, her respiratory function was increased, her pain was minimized, and her mental outlook was much stronger. She had made significant changes in her relationships and had addressed the root cause of her anger. The bare areas on the tongue had resolved and the pulses were stronger. The chest X-ray indicated that the mass was still there. At this point the patient felt she had the resources to undergo stem-cell treatments. The treatments went very well and the patient continued to use a range of naturopathic therapies to support her healing. In this situation the treatment intention initially was to manage the process, and then a radical intervention was chosen, followed by a treatment strategy that supported the healing process.

TYPE OF CHANGE REQUIRED

A practitioner determines the health risks, the degree of physiological change that has already occurred, and identifies the change that needs to occur in order to restore health. A practitioner often needs to clarify the difference between a patient's concern and the health risk of their disease. For example, a patient who has been diagnosed with liver cancer might not be in any discomfort but their health risks are high. A lot of change is needed immediately if the patient is to live. On the other hand, constant arthritic pain is very concerning and debilitating, but it is not a sign of high risk. When the health risks are low, treatments that are more gradual and gentle can be applied. When the health risks are high, treatments often are more dramatic and intense, if the goal is to restore health.

There are three main types of change that can occur: gradual, transitional, and transformational. Each one has its place and value in health care.

Gradual change

Results in improvements in lifestyle over time. If a patient is having mild symptoms and they make the necessary changes to their lifestyle and diet as the symptoms arise, these small changes will result in large benefits in the long term. Gradual change identifies and modifies the building blocks to health and addresses the lifestyle, external and environmental factors that can be improved over time to change the health outcome in the long run. Some examples include, increasing the amount and quality of fruits and vegetables that you eat, improving your breathing skills, exercising on a more regular basis, or spending more time relaxing and enjoying life. Gradual changes to health are ideal for health promotion and disease prevention strategies. Gradual changes are planned changes that involve a patient doing what they already do, but doing it 'better', for example, continually working to improve their nutrition and lifestyle. When the current health risks are low and there is a desire for long-term health, it is possible to consistently improve health by gradually introducing new health building strategies into your lifestyle. Gradual changes are gentle and they produce results that are more subtle and hence the challenge often comes in seeing the benefits and in maintaining the changes in the long run.

Transitional change

Is a shift from one state or behavior to another. The change at this level is more apparent. It involves adding, removing or modifying something specifically to impact health. For example, stopping dairy products completely to see if this improves chronic sinusitis, starting an exercise program to increase flexibility and cardiovascular function, learning the proper way to breathe and monitoring the improvement it has on anxiety or doing some mental exercises to address a situation that still triggers you. Transitional change is the most common type of change for patients who have health concerns or health risks that are bothersome but not currently life threatening. With transitional changes there is a period of time when the focus on a specific aspect of health or a specific energetic pattern is concentrated, the outcome is more immediate and a specific outcome is contributed to a specific change. Transitional change is also used when the aim of treatment is to improve quality of life and to decrease the rate of progression or spread of disease. If the changes address the root cause of the health concern, the body will return to and maintain a healthy state even after the change has been stopped.

Transformational change

Involves dramatic change and begins with a change in thinking. It is usually driven by a crisis such as when a patient is diagnosed with cancer or a serious illness. It is unplanned and involves changing a lot all at once. If a patient's intention is to survive a critical illness then it is necessary to assess all aspects of health and to make changes on all levels – psychological, functional, and structural. Changing diet and adding supplements often are not enough to restore health when faced with a serious disease. Transformation change addresses the root cause of disease, limits the triggers that are negatively affecting health, and supports the healing power of the body. Transformational change takes a lot of energy, focus, vitality, and will. It is through transformational changes that we see the true healing power of the body.

VITALITY AND WILL

The aim of most naturopathic treatments is to stimulate a patient's vital force. To do this you need to know the strength and ability of the body to heal and the progression of disease. The patient's will to live and their belief about life and death is also important. When the vitality and will is high, the ability of the patient to make dramatic changes is higher. If the vitality is low, it is important to support the body initially versus recommending or imposing changes that address this factor and a patient will not be able to handle.

> To evaluate vital force clinically, homeopaths synthesize their observations of a patient's appearance, verbal and nonverbal behaviors, resilience to daily hassles and major life events, personal medical status and history, family history, and capacity to live fully in joy and purpose (Bell et al 2004).

A practitioner's desire for health can never be stronger than the patient's. A practitioner is a guide. The patient needs to first determine their ultimate destination. There is a difference between quality of life and quantity. It is up to the patient to determine which one they desire. The desire for one over the other changes based on health concerns, age, and vitality. As perspectives change, practitioners have to be aware of these changes and provide treatments that support them. There is a difference between what medical science can do and what is appropriate to do for a specific individual.

CONSTITUTIONAL CONSIDERATIONS

A patient's energetic constitution provides insight into areas of susceptibility as well as into how a patient receives and processes information. Often the success and compliance of a treatment plan is influenced by how the information is conveyed and whether or not it is done in a manner that makes a patient feels comfortable.

- *Earth.* A person with an earth constitution is going to be more comfortable with specific details and with a structured plan. They often need to know what they are to do and why.
- *Water.* The relationship that is established with a water person is very important. They want to feel nurtured, listened to, and understood by the practitioner. It isn't so much the details, but how the treatment plan and communication flows.
- *Fire.* A fire person is going to be more comfortable when there is a specific focus and a direction to follow. A fire person needs to be motivated and enthusiastic about the changes and they do better with a few specific changes, not a whole list.
- *Air.* An air person will be most comfortable with choice. Provide a list for them to choose from or a range of activities that they can alternate between. Choice and variety are important to air persons.

TREATMENT CONSIDERATIONS

- Follow the principles of 'least force' and 'minimal dose'. Choose the most gentle treatment to achieve the desired effect.
- The body is a complex, dynamic system. Treatment might require addressing all aspects of an individual – the psychological, functional, and structural.

Treatment strategies

233

- Remember Hering's Law of Cure. Cure proceeds from above downward, from within outward, from the most important organs to least important organs, and expect symptoms to resolve in the reverse order of their appearance (Vithoulkas 1981)
- Address the building blocks to health; ensure the routes of elimination are functioning appropriately, and that the structure is aligned.
- No one is an island. When a patient makes changes, it impacts everyone in their support network. It is helpful to understand the impact that changes have on a patient's life.
- Communicate the assessment findings to your patient in a way that makes sense to them. Provide them with insight on what *they* need to do, what they need to change or focus on.
- It is what a patient does that determines the long lasting impact to health. Be cautious when patients 'outsource' their health; that is, when the primary effort of the patient is making and maintaining appointments.
- When you give a substance, the initial response represents the action of the substance in the body; subsequent responses represent the ability of the body to maintain the healing response or to handle the impact of that substance.
- Allow time for the body to adjust. Healing requires changes on many levels and this takes time. Anticipate the potential for a healing crisis and educate patients on the significance and benefit to the healing process.

REFERENCES

Bell IR et al 2004 Strength of vital force in classical homeopathy: bio-psycho-social-spiritual correlates within a complex systems context. J Altern Complement Med 10(1):123–131

McTaggart L 2002 The Field, The Quest for a Secret Force of the Universe. HarperCollins, London

Quinn JF 1996 The intention to heal: Perspectives of a therapeutic touch practitioner and researcher. Adv: J Mind-Body Health 12(3):26–30

Vithoulkas G 1981 The Science of Homeopathy. Grove Press, New York

FURTHER READING

Astin JA, Shapiro SL, Eisenberg DM, Forys KL 2003 Mind-body medicine: state of the science, implications for practice. J Am Board Fam Pract 16:131–147

Baron RJ 1985 An Introduction to medical phenomenology: I can't hear you while I'm listening. Ann Intern Med 103:606–611

Benor DJ 2006 Wholistic healing. The healing potential in a word – part III. Positive Health 12–13.

Lloyd IR 2006 Messages from the Body, a Guide to the Energetics of Health. Naturopathic Publications, Toronto

Magner LN 1992 A History of Medicine. Marcel Dekker, New York

DEFINITIONS

Acute healing response is an acute disease that has a rapid onset and a short course, resolving itself either by death, spontaneous recovery, or progressing to a chronic illness.

Aggravation refers to an increase in severity of symptoms; a worsening of symptoms or a disease state.

Allopathic is a term for standard Western medicine. The word comes from the Greek *allos* (different) and *pathein* (disease, suffering) and thus implying the use of drugs whose effects are different from those of the disease being treated.

Amplitude is the point of maximum intensity of the signal (usually regarded as the highest point on the wave).

Aspect refers to a particular feature, or situation. The position of something in relationship to something else, a part or component of something larger.

Ayurveda is a traditional system of medicine that is indigenous to India and been widely practiced for over 5000 years. The word Ayurveda is a Sanskrit term meaning 'science of life.' *Ayu* means 'life' or 'daily living' and *Veda* is 'knowing.' It deals with health in all its aspects: physical health, mental balance, spiritual well-being, social welfare, environmental considerations, dietary and lifestyle habits, daily living trends, and seasonal variations in lifestyle, as well as treating and managing specific diseases.

Balance is a state of equilibrium, a harmonious arrangement or relation of parts or elements within a whole.

Biomedical model is based on anatomical and physiological observation. It is the view the body is organized into a variety of systems (cardiovascular, respiratory, urinary, etc.) controlled by corresponding organs (heart, lungs, kidney, etc.)

Body refers to the functional and structural aspects of an individual.

Cause relates to the event that is responsible for an effect, result, or consequence, such as the fundamental cause of disease.

Causality is the interrelation of cause and effect.

Chinese medicine (CM) is a traditional system of health care from China that has been practiced for over 3000 years. CM is based on a concept of balanced Qi (pronounced 'chee'), or vital energy, that is believed to flow throughout the body. Disease is proposed to result from the flow of Qi being disrupted and Yin and Yang becoming imbalanced. Among the components of CM are herbal and nutritional therapy, restorative physical exercises, meditation, acupuncture, and remedial massage.

Chiropractic medicine is an alternative discipline that views the spine as the backbone of human health. Misalignments of vertebrae caused by poor posture or trauma cause pressure on the spinal nerve roots, leading to diminished function and illness. Through manipulation or adjustment of the spine, treatment seeks to analyze and correct misalignments.

Coherence is the consistency between different aspects of an individual. It refers to the physical congruity and consistency of aspects of the body marked by when electromagnetic waves are in-phase.

Collective consciousness is the shared beliefs and moral attitudes which operate as a unifying force within society.

Complementary and alternative medicine (CAM) is a group of diverse medical and health care systems, practices, and products that are not presently considered an integral part of conventional medicine.

Constitution is the inherent and natural state of an individual. The unique energetic composition or makeup of a person, the way in which someone or something is composed. The physical body and mental temperament that is expressive of the natural traits and predisposition of the individual.

Conventional medicine is a whole medical system practiced by medical doctors and by their allied health professionals, such as physical therapists, psychologists, and registered nurses. Other terms for conventional medicine include allopathy; Western, mainstream, and orthodox medicine; and biomedicine.

Cure means to restore to health, to make whole again, through curative means or through the natural process of healing. It is the restoration of health.

Disease is a state of disharmony or lack of coherence between or among different aspects of an individual. It is a state of health or well being that is different than what is desired.

Doshas is a term used in Ayurvedic medicine that literally means 'fault' or 'mistake'. A dosha is one of the three forces which bind the five elements down into living flesh and that determines an individual's constitution. The three doshas are vata, pitta, and kapha.

Dualism refers to the separation of mind and body.

Eastern medicine is a broad term for Oriental, Indian, Tibetan, Japanese, and Chinese medicine, all of which share philosophies about the energy system of the human body and the necessity of balance and harmony.

Electromagnetic fields (EMFs, also called electric and magnetic fields) refer to the invisible lines of force that surround all electrical devices. The Earth also produces EMFs; electric fields are produced when there is thunderstorm activity, and magnetic fields are believed to be produced by electric currents flowing from the Earth's core.

Elements refers to the substances of traditional medicine, such as ether, air, fire, water, and earth. These substances are believed to constitute all aspects of the universe.

Energetic shift relates to a change in the pattern of energetic manifestation. Energy shifts in response to all influences that it encounters. Whether the energetic shift is toward health or toward disease depends on a number of interacting factors.

Energy is a foundational aspect of life. It refers to the electromagnetic wave patterns that surround every aspect of life. It is the vibrational quality of a substance that is responsible for communication and movement.

Essence is the attribute (or set of attributes) that make an object or substance what it fundamentally is, and that it has necessarily (in contrast with accidental properties that the object or substance has contingently, and without which the substance could not have existed). Essence is the whole of oneself and includes the subjective as well as objective.

Frequency is a rate of oscillation measured by the number of wave cycles per unit time (usually in cycles per second, or hertz).

Gunas is an Ayurvedic term that describes the three basic qualities of Nature that determine the inherent characteristics of all created things. The gunas are sattva (purity, light, harmony, intelligence); rajas (activity, passion); and tamas (dullness, inertia, ignorance).

Harmony is the orderly relationship of all parts working together.

Health is the harmonious vibration of the psychological, functional, and structural aspects of an individual with their personal essence and their external environment. Health is the freedom from disease or abnormality, a condition of optimal well-being or functioning.

Heterostasis is a disease state.

Holistic or *holism* means all, entire, or total. It is based on the belief that the whole is greater than the sum of the parts. When assessing human beings, it refers to the consideration of the spiritual, psychological, functional, and structural aspects of an individual, as well as the environmental and social factors.

Homeodynamic state is a state of health, the inherent ability of the body to maintain a relatively constant internal environment.

Homeopathic medicine is an alternative medical system. The term *homeopathy* derives from the Greek *homoion pathos*, which means 'similar suffering'. By comparison, the term *allopathy* which refers to orthodox (conventional) medicine, comes from *allos*, meaning 'different'. In homeopathic medicine, there is a belief that 'like cures like,' meaning that small, highly diluted quantities of medicinal substances are given to cure symptoms, when the same substances given at higher or more concentrated doses would actually cause those symptoms.

Homeostasis refers to a state of health. This is an old term, refer to homeodynamic state.

Humor refers to the temperament or disposition of an individual.

Individual relates to the combination of the psychological, functional, and structural aspects of a person, as a unit.

Influence refers to the power to produce an effect on someone or something by imperceptible or intangible means.

Interactionism is the study of the communication and relationship between biophysical and psychosocial mechanisms and aspects of life.

Law of similars is the principle that 'like shall be cured by like' that forms the basis of homeopathy; the proper remedy for a patient's disease is that substance that is capable of producing, in a healthy person, symptoms similar to those from which the patient suffers.

Life force is the force, power, or energy which enlivens the material organism. In health, the spirit-like life force that enlivens the material organism as dynamic, governs without restriction and keeps all parts of the organism in admirable, harmonious, vital operation.

Linear causality is based on a direct relationship between one cause and one effect.

Mechanism treats Nature, including living systems, as machinery, obeying fixed laws and tending to explain phenomena only by reference to physical or biological causes and tangible parts.

Mutual causality denotes a relationship between one event (cause) and another event (effect) which is the consequence of the first. With mutual causality similar conditions might produce dissimilar results based on the involvement of external factors and internal feedback influences.

Osteopathic medicine is a form of conventional medicine that has an underlying belief that all of the body's systems work together, and disturbances in one system may affect function elsewhere in the body. Some osteopathic physicians practice osteopathic manipulation, a full-body system of hands-on techniques to alleviate pain, restore function, and promote health and well-being.

Peak is the highest point on a wave.

Polarity therapy is an alternative system of health based on philosophies of Chinese and Ayurvedic medicine. It uses diet and hands-on therapy to balance the electromagnetic energy of an individual and to enhance overall health and wellbeing.

Prana is the life force, equivalent to the Qi in oriental medicine; the vital life-sustaining force of both the body and the universe.

Qi is a Chinese term for vital energy or life force. In traditional Chinese medicine, Qi is believed to regulate a person's spiritual, emotional, mental, and physical balance, and to be influenced by the opposing forces of yin and yang. The concept of Qi, or some similar vital force, is incorporated into many therapies used in the holistic approach to health.

Reductionism asserts that the nature of complex things can be explained and broken down into smaller parts and sums of simpler or more fundamental things.

Root cause is the factor or factors that initiated a shift away from a healthy state.

Self-organization is a characteristic of complex systems and it relates to the ability of systems to maintain a complex pattern of organization.

Self-renewal is the ability of living systems to continuously renew and recycle their components while maintaining the integrity of their overall structure.

Signals refers to the stimulus that is responsible for initiating cellular communication.

Susceptibility represents an individual's tendencies, both their strengths and their weaknesses.

Symptom is a bodily sensation experienced by a patient which indicates a shift away from health.

Systems theory is a set of related definitions, assumptions and propositions that deal with reality as an integrated hierarchy of matter and energy. It studies the nature of complex systems in nature, society, and science. It is a framework by which one can analyze and/or describe any group of objects that work in concert to produce some result.

Traditional medicine describes medical systems which developed over centuries within various societies before the era of modern medicine. Traditional medicine includes the practices of Ayurvedic, Chinese, and Unani medicine.

Trough is the lowest point of a wave.

Unani medicine is a traditional Greek system of medicine that as been practiced in India, Persia, Pakistan and other countries for thousands of years. It is based on the theory that everything in the universe is comprised of four temperaments that have the qualities of heat, moistness, coldness, and dryness. Unani medicine recognizes that health and disease have mental, emotional, spiritual, and physical causes. It also believes that each individual should take responsibility for their own well-being and that the body has an innate power to heal.

Vitalism is the view that life is governed by forces beyond oneself. These forces are unique to living beings and permit them to go on living. The forces cannot be reduced to physical laws. Often it is associated with notions of spirit or soul.

Vitality refers to the inherent capacity of an organism to live, grow, develop, and heal.

Wave is a movement of energy around a directional axis.

Wavelength is the length or distance between two identical points on the wave (which comprises one complete wave cycle). This is described with different terms of measurement, depending on the size of the wave.

Western medicine a term used to describe allopathic medicine, orthodox medicine, or the way medicine has been practiced in the United States and Europe. Pharmaceutical products and surgery are the major modalities used to combat disease.

Yin–Yang is a Chinese concept that describes all existence in terms of states or conditions that are different but mutually dependent; traditional Chinese medicine aims to restore balance to these contrasting aspects.

Definitions

INDEX

Please note that page references relating to non-textual content such as Figures or Tables are in *italic* print

Index

Index

Printed in the United States
By Bookmasters